"Man, by his actions, sets into motion those agencies which can eventually destroy him".
— *Pythagoras (c. 597–504* B.C.*)*

Guidebook to Nutritional Factors in Foods

By David A. Phillips, Ph.D., N.D., B.E.

Published by
Woodbridge Press Publishing Company
Santa Barbara, California 93111

Published by

Woodbridge Press Publishing Company
Post Office Box 6189
Santa Barbara, California 93111

Copyright © 1979, 1977 by David A. Phillips

Library of Congress Catalog Card Number: 79-10010

International Standard Book Number: 0-912800-71-2

Published simultaneously in the United States and Canada

Printed in the United States of America

Library of Congress Cataloging in Publication Data

Phillips, David A
    Guidebook to nutritional factors in foods.

    Edition of 1977 published under title: Guide book to nutritional factors in edible foods.
    1. Food—Composition—Tables.   I. Title.
TX551.P517   1979   641.1   79-10010
ISBN 0-912800-71-2

*This book is dedicated to the improved health,
more enjoyable eating and happier life of
every citizen of this world.*

*David A. Phillips,
104 Bowden Street,
West Ryde, 2114,
Australia.*

Acknowledgements

For their helpfulness and co-operation, the following companies and organizations are given special thanks by this author:

American Maple Products Corporation, Newport, Vermont
Covalda Date Company, Coachella, California
Norganic Foods Company, Anaheim, California
Rodale Press, Emmaus, Pennsylvania
United States Department of Agriculture, Washington, D.C.

The following organizations in Australia and New Zealand:

Brancourts Pty. Ltd.; Bread Research Institute; Commonwealth Department of Health; C.S.I.R.O. Division of Food Research; CSR Company Limited; Gillespie Bros. Pty. Ltd.; Healtheries of New Zealand Ltd.; Hygienic Food Supplies Pty. Ltd.; Oliveholme Limited; Public Library of N.S.W.; Ricegrowers Co-operative Mills Ltd.; San Remo Macaroni Co. Pty. Ltd.

Contents

SECTION ONE

Your Guide to a Better Diet 9

Components 10; Comparisons 11

Average Daily Nutritional Requirements 13

General 13; Zinc 15; Manganese 15; Iodine 15;
Copper 16; Pantothenic acid 16; Vitamin B₆ 16;
Vitamin B₁₂ and Biotin 16; Folic acid 16;
Vitamin D 17; Vitamin E 17

SECTION TWO

Nutritional Factors

Abbreviations 23; Averages 24; Boiled vegetables 24;
Dried fruits 25; Food juices 26; Meats 26; Oxalic acid 26;
Sprouts 27; Sweeteners 28

Food Nutrient Tables 29

SECTION THREE

Guidance with Certain Foods 45

Avocados 46; Beef 46; Bread 47; Bulghur Wheat 47;
Buttermilk 48; Cabbage 48; Carob 48; Cheeses 49;
Coconut 49; Cornflakes 50; Eggs 50; Figs, dried 51;
Gluten flour 51; Liver 52; Maple 52; Milks 53; Miso 54;
Pasta 54; Rice 55; Sesame seeds 55; Soya beans 55;
Soya grits 56; Soya milk 56; T.V.P. 57; Vinegars 57;
Yogurt 58

SECTION FOUR

Protein   59

   Table: Protein content of foods 62
   Table: Major nutrients in protein-rich foods 64

Fat   67

   Tables: Fat content of foods 69, 70

Fatty Acids and Cholesterol   72

   Table: Fatty acid and cholesterol content of foods 76

Edible Oils   79

   Extraction 79; Bottling 80; Processing 81

Food Energy–Calories   83

   Tables: Food energy available from foods 86, 88

Total Carbohydrates   91

Fiber   93

   Tables: Total carbohydrates in foods 96, 98
   Table: Fiber content of foods 100

Minerals   101

   Tables: Calcium content of foods 104
           Phosphorous content of foods 106
           Iron content of foods 108
           Sodium content of foods 110
           Potassium content of foods 112
           Magnesium content of foods 114

Vitamins   116

  Tables: Vitamin A content of foods 119
         Vitamin B_1 content of foods 120
         Vitamin B_2 content of foods 122
         Vitamin B_3—niacin—content of foods 124
         Vitamin C content of foods 126

Additional Reading and Reference   128

Your Guide to a Better Diet

This book is the outcome of years of research and considerable co-operation from many people and organisations. It is designed to be used as a basic guide to understanding the nutritional values of foods available for consumption in U.S.A., Australia and other Western Countries.

This series of food facts and figures is intended to assist in satisfying the much needed basis for nutritional and health awareness in our present education system. It is a fundamental basis to human welfare to realise that diet and health are intimately related. The only sound way to build the basis for permanent good health is through a nutritious diet. And what better way is there to obtain a nutritious diet than to be aware of the nutritional components of our foods?

This book is designed for every person who eats food. Whether one's interest be motivated by flavors, facts or fancies, the following nutritional information is very important and is arranged for easy understanding. Special benefits will be conferred upon dieticians, nutritionists and all healing practitioners who make use of these analyses. As well, the use of this book will considerably benefit housewives, sportspeople, businessmen (especially their secretaries), people seeking to lose weight or to gain weight, those with vitamin or mineral deficiencies; in fact, by every thinking person who seeks to improve his or her health, fitness and figure by the greatest single influence — food.

Components

The composition of the modern diet is impossible to itemise briefly. Western Society is composed of many different ethnic and cultural groups, most of which have introduced particular dietary habits. These have been largely modified by the Industrial Revolution and its resultant "convenience factor" which gives preference to filling the stomach, rather than nourishing the body. This has more recently given rise to the formation of many health-oriented associations whose members especially demand to know more about the components of their diet.

Of special influence on today's dietary pattern is the New Age generation. Thinking young people recognise the need for more natural living and the necessity of basing their diets upon whole, unprocessed foods. They seek freedom from illness and incapacity and they know diet to be fundamental to this.

With such a broad base upon which to propound a list of components in the modern diet, it early became apparent that a book which contained every aspect of each individual food would grow to many hundreds of pages. This would somewhat defeat the author's basic intent of providing a succinct, ready-reference guide to food nutrients.

The compromise was reached with this offering. The reasons for particular inclusions or omissions are discussed further on. In general, the components of this book are those foods which are grown or prepared in the U.S.A., Canada, Australia, Europe and South Africa. Every endeavor has been made to include adequate representation of every food group, with greatest coverage directed towards natural foods.

Comparisons

A most essential feature of the nutritional values of edible foods is a table of clear comparisons for as many nutrients as scientific research has been able to isolate in the laboratory. Such a comprehensive table then forms a basis for the extraction of graduated lists of each food within a nutrient group. This provides a direct comparison for recognising the foods which are abundant in any particular nutrient.

Sets of comprehensive, graduated nutrient values of edible foods are a special feature of this book and a most vital guide to all health-oriented, diet-conscious people.

There are twenty such sets of graduated tables in the following pages, most of which are arranged in descending order of nutrient concentration. Three exceptions are for fats, calories and total carbohydrates, where for each a second graduated list has been tabulated in ascending order — from the lowest concentrations upwards — as a special guide to people seeking minimal amounts of these factors in their diets.

It will be seen that the first set of tables is the general, comprehensive listing of food compositions from which particular direct comparisons can be readily made for different types of breads, cheeses, flours, milks and yeasts, all of which are grouped conveniently together. Direct comparisons can also be made for each fruit and vegetable in its varied states of preparation — between raw and boiled or juiced or sprouted/or dried, etc. It must be realised that, in every case, the figures quoted are averages for each food, as explained in Section Two.

Average
Daily Nutritional
Requirements

The following table of human nutritional requirements is offered as a general and an average guide to suitable diet selection. This will be found of considerable assistance when used in conjunction with the nutrient tables given in this book, especially to those who are on a restricted diet or who have weight control problems.

Dietary needs of people can vary quite considerably between males and females, between people of different age groups, body structures and emotional dispositions, between those living in different climatic areas, involved in different occupations, etc. Therefore, to provide a comprehensive list of dietary nutritional requirements for all possibilities would create a mass of figures which would frighten all but the professional nutritionist. As this book is intended to be a guide to everyone, it was decided to employ a basic nine occupational and age variation groups.

Figures quoted on the accompanying nutrient table represent the results of latest research carried out by this author and many other practicing nutritionists. In some instances, the figures are consistent with those recommended by the National Academy of Sciences; but variations resulting from practical experience contribute to making this table the most reliable offered in any dietary guidebook yet published.

Nutritional requirements for people employed in hard, manual work (male or female), sportsmen and sportswomen, as well as for those in more advanced years living a physically quiet life or those who are convalescing from illness, all vary quite significantly in their requirements of most nutrients, compared with the average requirements of adults. The nutritional requirements of pregnant or lactating women also vary from those of most other women. This author has always lamented the lack of such specific guidance in other publications of a similar nature.

Again, in terms of comprehensiveness, this nutrient table appears to exceed all thus far in print in its provision of guidelines for the intakes of as many as 25 different nutrients. This is currently the maximum number of which it is possible to research for the daily requirements. Of these 25 nutrients, comprehensive food sources can now be tabulated for 14, as shown in the following pages. Of the remaining 11 nutrients, insufficient research has thus far been completed to provide detailed tables of food sources. However, we do know the general types of foods in which these eleven nutrients are found to be most abundant. They are as follows:

Zinc

Most abundant in protein-rich foods: *viz.,* nuts, seeds, meats, fish, egg yolks, poultry and brewers yeast; also in whole grains, dairy products, yellow and green vegetables (especially carrots, corn and peas) and yellow fruits, such as papayas and mangoes. Zinc is noticeably deficient in processed foods, especially packaged and processed cereals.

Manganese

The richest source is wheat germ. Whole grains are especially good sources, especially wheat, oats and rye. Most vegetables contain small but important quantities of manganese.

Iodine

All sea foods are naturally the most prolific sources, especially cod liver oil. Important vegetable sources are dried beans, asparagus and all green vegetables.

Copper

Found in all nuts and all dried peas and beans. Also found in animal livers, wheat bran, whole wheat, molasses, dried currants, mushrooms, broccoli and avocadoes.

Pantothenic Acid

Brewers and torula yeast, liver and other animal organ meats, wheat and rice brans, wheat germ, peanuts, sesame seeds, legumes, soya beans, eggs and buckwheat.

Vitamin B6

Brewers and torula yeast, rice bran, wheat germ, all whole grains, all beans, liver, chicken, most fish, corn and peanut oils, bananas, walnuts, peanuts, cabbages, beets, oranges, lemons and corn.

Vitamin B12 and Biotin

Same food sources as vitamins B_1, B_2 and B_3.

Folic Acid

Wheat germ and bran, all beans and legumes, animal organ meats, green vegetables (especially asparagus), mushrooms, potatoes and oranges.

Vitamin D

By far the best source is **unobstructed** sunlight. Food sources are cod liver oil, egg yolk, salmon and tuna fish.

Vitamin E

The most abundant natural sources are wheat and rice germs; then, to a much lesser degree, wheat and other whole grains, green leafy vegetables, nuts and legumes.

AVERAGE DAILY

	PROTEIN - grams	FOOD ENERGY - calories	FIBER - grams	CALCIUM - milligrams	PHOSPHORUS - milligrams	IRON - milligrams	SODIUM - grams	POTASSIUM - milligrams	MAGNESIUM - milligrams
Infants (to 1 year)	5-10	1000	.5	300	150	1	.14	500	40
Children (1 – 12 yrs)	20-30	1500-2500	2-4	600-1000	400-1000	3-10	.2	1000-1500	100-200
Youths (13–19yrs)	40-60	3500	5	1300	1300	15	.4	2500	350
Men	50	3000	5	1000	1000	12	.5	3000	400
Women	40	2200	5	800	800	14	.5	2500	350
Manual Workers	60	4000	5	1100	1100	12	.5	3500	500
Sports People	80	4500	5	1200	1200	14	.6	4000	600
Pregnant & Lactating Women	50	2600	5	1500	1300	16	.6	3000	450
Retired & Convalescent People	35	2000	5	1000	1000	10	.4	2000	300

NUTRITIONAL REQUIREMENTS

ZINC - milligrams	MANGANESE - milligrams	IODINE - milligrams	COPPER - milligrams	VITAMIN A - milligrams	VITAMIN B_1 - milligrams	VITAMIN B_2 - milligrams	VITAMIN B_3 - milligrams	PANTOTHENIC ACID - milligrams	VITAMIN B_6 - milligrams	VITAMIN B_{12} - micrograms	FOLIC ACID - milligrams	BIOTIN - milligrams	VITAMIN C - milligrams	VITAMIN D - international units	VITAMIN E - international units
4	1	.04	.5	.4	.2	.4	2	2	.4	2	.1	.05	40	400	5
6-8	3-15	.10	1	.6-1.0	.5-1.0	.6-1.2	6-16	3-6	.7-2	3-4	.2-.4	.1-.2	50-80	400	8-14
15	20	.15	2	1.5	1.8	2.5	20	8	5	6	.6	.3	100	400	20
15	25	.18	2	1.5	1.5	1.8	18	10	4	6	.5	.3	75	400	30
15	20	.15	2	1.2	1.3	1.6	15	10	3	6	.5	.3	75	400	25
18	28	.22	2	1.5	1.7	2.0	20	10	4	6	.5	.3	100	400	40
20	30	.30	2	1.8	2.0	2.7	22	12	5	7	.6	.3	150	400	50
25	25	.18	2	2.4	1.8	2.5	18	10	4	8	.8	.3	150	400	30
20	18	.14	2	1.5	1.3	1.8	15	8	3	5	.5	.3	100	400	40

Nutritional Factors

The following sets of nutritional tables contain only those food factors which are generally accepted as nutrients and have been analysed in a sufficient number of foods to provide adequate, reliable comparisons. Water contents in all foods have been also included as these are vital to the total understanding of a food's composition and for those people who wish to compare nutrients in different foods.

Until recent years, food analysis tables included up to only five mineral elements. Recent important research on the magnesium content of foods has embraced a sufficient number of different items to encourage its inclusion in our general table as a sixth mineral element. It is to be hoped that continued research will soon provide us with similar details of other mineral and vitamin components in a sufficiently comprehensive manner to permit their inclusion in subsequent editions of this book.

Already we know of dozens more mineral elements and vitamins included in many foods, but not yet the subject of sufficient analysis to provide a comprehensive pattern for tabulation. It is not unreasonable to assume that many more such nutritional factors await discovery or confirmation. In fact it is quite probable that science will never be able to totally uncover every nutritional factor in foods or the extent to which each such factor relates to the others or functions in human dietetics.

Recognising nutrition in its broadest sense, we see that certain vital aspects of a food's nutritional properties have not yet lent themselves to reliable tabulation. These factors are of a more metaphysical (beyond physical measurement) nature and are generally and conveniently referred to as a food's "life force." Some scientists and health practitioners have ridiculed the premise that such components of foods could possibly exist. As a lecturer and consultant in nutrition for many years, this author has met many such skeptics. However, the last few years have witnessed a noticeable decline in the opposition to such recognition. This is not surprising in the face of the increasing flow of more and more documented evidence in support of the vital role of a food's life force components especially where fresh raw foods have been therapeutically used with great success in overcoming hitherto "incurable" diseases such as arthritis and cancer.

Some recent best-selling books testifying to the feelings of plants and related metaphysical aspects of a botanical nature indicate that a new branch of nutritional research is about to emerge. This will throw an important light onto the subject of nutrition and provide a valuable guide to such hitherto inexplicable conditions as why a nutrient-rich food might create indigestion, why a nutrient-poor food can provide such surprising satisfaction, etc.

Although the chemical analyses of foods provide something a little short of the total nutritional picture, they are at least an excellent basis for preparing the picture. They are, in fact, the only factors we have available for guidance and comparison at this time.

Some general explanations will assist the reader to gain a more accurate understanding of nutritional factors in foods listed in this book:

Abbreviations

Two frequent abbreviations are used throughout the tables.

NA — Not Available. When used in place of a nutritional value, this indicates that a reliable figure is not currently available. In most cases, insufficient verifiable research has been undertaken on this factor in foods.

Tr — Trace. This abbreviation indicates that the nutrient in question is present only as a trace amount, analysed to be a figure less than that showing as the minimum for any food in that nutritional column.

Averages

All figures quoted for each nutrient must represent averages of analysed samples. Such samples are generally typical of the range available on the open market, an average allowing for variations in methods of agriculture, time of harvest, manner of storage, degree of manufacture and recipe used, etc. It is especially important to note that fresh foods available on the open market are generally cultivated by modern, chemically-based techniques. Foods which are produced by organic or biodynamic methods, free from chemical enforcement or sprays, are known to develop higher levels in all nutrients, except starches: these are held in check. For documentation and further explanation on this subject, refer this author's health book, *From Soil To Psyche.**

Boiled Vegetables

Analysts generally prefer the use of boiled vegetables for obtaining their nutritional values for the cooked state. In a sense, this is helpful to nutritionists, as boiling usually causes the greatest nutritional losses in cooking, thereby highlighting the advantage of eating raw foods. (This important aspect of diet is also detailed in *From Soil To Psyche*.) A far better method of cooking is steaming. This significantly reduces the nutrient loss in cooking, especially of water-soluble minerals and vitamins, as well as the natural sugars. Cooking is primarily intended to render certain vegetables softer — the more easily chewed and digested. This is defeated if a

*From Soil To Psyche is published by Woodbridge Press, Santa Barbara, California.

major loss of nutrients and of flavor is created, as when boiling is undertaken. Steaming is the means of holding vegetables above the level of the boiling water, best facilitated by the use of a stainless steel, flexible, perforated steamer stand. But be sure it is totally stainless steel and guaranteed, such as the VITA-SAVER, available throughout U.S.A., Australia, and Canada. Cheaper Asian-made imitations use inferior steel and often employ aluminium legs to reduce costs. Aluminium cookware has been repeatedly proven greatly inferior to stainless steel, as well as being potentially toxic to cooked foods.

Dried Fruits

Many fruits are dried to facilitate their storage for extended periods and to allow them to be the most easily transported. Drying is an age-old method of preservation which originally depended on the heat of the sun. Today, we recognise the advantages of sun-drying fruits, such as dates, figs, apricots and other stone fruits, especially when compared to the modern methods of faster, chemical drying. It was discovered that when sulphur was burned in the presence of drying fruits, they achieved a lighter color and dried more quickly, especially when dehydrated in ovens. Sulphur-drying precipitates sulphur dioxide (SO_2) on the surface of fruits and, when this combines with water in the body, forms sulphurous acid (H_2SO_3), a kidney irritant when ingested in sufficient quantities. The reduced flavors of sulphur-dried fruits suggest that the extra time demanded by sun-drying is a many-fold investment, natural flavors being a general indication of nutritional properties. Certain fruits, such as bananas and pineapples, do not successfully sun dry and need the higher temperatures of dehydration ovens (140°F) to facilitate proper drying.

Food Juices

Observation of the nutrient tables will reveal that when fruits or vegetables are juiced, their nutritional values are often reduced. For the body's optimum nutritional requirements, it is obvious that the whole food should be eaten. However, if drinking is demanded, the consumption of fruit or vegetable juices will provide one of the highest level of nutrients available from any form of drink. It is always best to juice vegetables and fruits freshly for immediate drinking, rather than storing them or buying canned or preserved juices, all of which have been cooked as part of their processing.

Meats

Due to the huge variety of cuts and types of meats available, only a representative selection has been chosen for this book. This selection will be seen to include animal flesh meats, liver, preserved meats, seafood and poultry. Such items can be taken as a general guide to the nutritional properties of similar cuts or varieties of meat not shown.

Oxalic Acid

Certain foodstuffs possess levels of oxalic acid such as to demand of them special mention. Oxalic acid is an acute irritant to the kidneys, so the body ensures that it is handled in the least harmful manner by having it combine with calcium and magnesium to form oxalates — salts with a sharp crystal formation. These are often the foundation of kidney stones if unduly abundant in the area. Such pathological implications are beyond our immediate consideration. However, it is important to note that oxalic acid in foods is responsible for the effective reduction of calcium and magnesium levels in those foods, or the reduction of their reserves within the body. For this reason, it is important to take care of the quantity of foods ingested when it is known that they are possessors of oxalic acid. The most commonly-consumed substances containing significant concentrations of oxalic acid are tea, coffee and cocoa (chocolate), then meat, beet greens, spinach, and rhubarb. Most nuts contain smaller amounts of oxalic acid, but these are no problem to the body, as nuts contain more than adequate calcium.

Sprouts

Reliable analyses are available only for mung bean and soya bean sprouts, yet from the comparisons of these with the standard dry mung beans and soya beans, it is obvious how the nutrient increase from sprouting makes this a very valuable method of food preparation. To obtain an accurate comparison of nutrients between the sprouted and dry beans, it is necessary to first relate the water contents to obtain the same basis. This is done in detail in *From Soil To Psyche*, where it is shown how spectacularly certain nutrients increase when sprouting takes place. Other foods suited to sprouting include most grains, beans, lentils and seeds.

Sweeteners

Most people have come to conventionally accept refined sugar as the most convenient manner for sweetening foods and drinks. However, they fail to take into account that beet and cane sugar crystals possess only very minimal nutrients when in the raw or brown state, and virtually no nutrients when refined. To facilitate its digestion, sugar must deplete the body's stores of nutrients. Added to this leaching factor, the digestion of cane or beet sugars imposes a highly acidic residual in the mouth, predisposing towards a great risk of dental caries. Honey is a more acceptable alternative to the body. However, its concentrated sweetness also tends to deplete the body's insulin store by almost as much as sugar. Carob powder is by far one of the best natural sweeteners; as the tables reveal, it contains a high level of many nutrients. However, carob is far less sweet than sugar and does not suit all uses. The final alternative is maple sugar, as discussed in the following Section. Although far more expensive than standard sugar, maple is also a food, the sweetest known to man.

Food Nutrient Tables...

FOOD NUTRIENT TABLES

FOOD	Water	Protein	Fat	Food Energy	Total Carbo-hydrates	Fibre	Calcium
per 100g edible portion	g	g	g	Calories	g	g	mg
Almond kernels — natural, raw	5	19.5	53.8	598	18.9	2.6	245
Apples — with peel, raw	84	.3	.6	57	14.2	1.0	7
— peeled, raw	85	.3	.3	53	13.8	.6	6
— dried	21	1.3	1.6	289	75.2	3.1	27
juice — canned	88	.1	Tr	42	11.5	.1	6
Apricots — raw	.86	.8	.2	45	11.4	.6	16
— dried	24	4.5	.4	265	68.3	3.0	84
nectar — canned	85	.3	.1	57	14.6	.2	9
Artichokes, Globe — raw	86	2.9	.2	40	10.6	2.4	51
— boiled	87	2.8	.2	37	9.9	2.4	51
Jerusalem — raw	80	1.9	.1	68	16.7	.8	26
Asparagus — raw	93	2.1	.2	21	3.8	.7	23
— boiled	94	1.9	.2	20	3.6	.7	20
Avocadoes — Average all varieties	75	1.7	15.8	161	6.3	1.6	12
— Fuerte variety	74	2.2	17.0	171	6.0	1.5	12
Bacon — grilled	10	27.2	59.3	661	2.7	0	29
Bananas — ripe, raw	75	1.1	.3	87	22.5	.5	9
— dehydrated	3	4.4	.8	340	88.6	2.0	32
Barley — pearled, dry	11	7.9	1.7	354	79.1	.5	12
Beans (long green) — raw	91	1.8	.2	32	6.8	1.0	48
— boiled	90	1.7	.2	30	6.4	1.0	46
Beef Steak (T-bone) — "rare"	59	21.5	18.5	258	0	0	16
— "well done"	33	33.1	32.9	437	0	0	23
Beet Greens — raw	91	2.2	.3	24	4.6	1.3	119
— boiled	94	1.7	.2	18	3.3	1.1	99
Beets — raw	88	1.6	.1	40	9.3	.8	26
— boiled	91	1.1	.1	31	7.0	.8	21
Bell Peppers — raw	93	1.2	.2	26	5.6	1.5	10
Blackberries — raw	84	1.2	1.0	58	12.7	4.1	41
Brazil Nut kernels — raw	5	14.3	66.9	654	10.9	3.1	186
Bread							
— Brown (50% wholemeal/white)	39	8.0	1.8	242	49.1	.8	20
— Cracked Wheat	40	8.5	2.5	235	46.7	1.3	35
— Dark Rye (added molasses)	40	7.6	1.5	237	48.8	.9	62
— Light Rye (30% rye, 70% wheat)	40	7.6	1.5	238	49.1	1.1	75
— Mixed Grain	38	9.2	2.8	240	48.0	.9	NA
— White Wheat	39	7.8	1.5	243	49.9	.2	14
— Wholemeal (Wheat)	40	8.1	2.4	230	46.7	1.3	35
Breadfruit — raw	70	1.7	.3	106	25.2	1.2	33
Bream fish — steamed	77	17.8	3.0	101	0	0	35
Broadbeans — fresh, raw	72	8.4	.4	105	17.8	2.2	27
— dry, raw	12	25.1	1.7	338	58.2	6.7	102
Broccoli — raw	88	3.6	.3	35	6.3	1.5	123
— boiled	91	3.1	.3	26	4.9	1.5	98

Phos-phorus	Iron	Sodium	Potassium	Magnes-ium	Vitamin A	Vitamin B1 Thiamine	Vitamin B2 Ribo-flavin	Vitamin B3 Niacin	Vitamin C Ascorbic Acid
mg	mg	mg	mg	mg	mg	mg	mg	mg	mg
473	4.3	4	773	270	0	.24	.75	3.6	9
9	.3	2	115	NA	.01	.04	.03	.2	10
9	.3	2	115	5	Tr	.04	.03	.2	6
52	1.7	5	569	22	Tr	.08	.11	.8	10
9	.3	2	106	4	0	.01	.02	.1	1
23	.5	2	294	12	.25	.03	.05	.8	8
114	4.3	23	1,561	62	.88	.01	.17	3.2	10
12	.2	Tr	151	NA	.10	.01	.01	.2	3
88	1.3	43	430	NA	.02	.08	.05	1.0	12
69	1.1	30	301	NA	.02	.07	.04	.7	8
78	.5	3	420	11	Tr	.20	.04	.7	6
62	1.0	3	241	20	.09	.16	.19	1.4	33
51	.8	1	183	NA	.09	.15	.18	1.3	25
34	.6	4	455	45	.03	.09	.21	1.5	13
42	.6	4	604	45	.03	.11	.20	1.6	14
292	2.7	3,328	462	25	0	.50	.31	5.1	0
27	.6	1	377	33	.03	.06	.05	.7	11
104	2.8	4	1,477	132	.12	.18	.24	2.8	7
228	1.1	3	141	37	0	.12	.07	1.6	0
46	.8	5	272	32	.06	.08	.10	.5	21
44	.8	5	258	NA	.06	.06	.07	.4	12
209	3.3	82	377	21	.01	.06	.16	4.3	0
322	5.0	126	580	NA	.02	.10	.25	6.7	0
40	3.3	130	570	106	.69	.10	.22	.4	30
25	1.9	76	332	NA	.58	.07	.15	.3	15
38	.8	78	320	25	Tr	.03	.05	.3	10
29	.6	52	201	15	Tr	.03	.04	.3	6
30	.6	8	216	18	.06	.05	.07	.4	231
22	.9	2	171	30	.03	.03	.04	.4	22
693	3.4	1	715	225	Tr	.96	.12	1.6	0
NA	1.7	538	252	NA	Tr	.21	.11	2.4	0
NA	3.0	529	204	35	0	.27	.09	2.6	0
124	1.6	593	159	71	0	.20	.06	1.0	0
147	1.6	557	145	42	0	.17	.07	1.4	0
NA	NA	NA	NA	NA	0	NA	NA	NA	0
74	1.0	507	85	22	0	.13	.08	.9	0
NA	3.0	529	204	78	0	.27	.09	2.6	0
32	1.2	15	439	NA	.01	.11	.03	.9	29
238	.6	113	281	NA	Tr	.06	.10	3.0	Tr
157	2.2	4	471	NA	.03	.28	.17	1.6	30
391	7.1	10	NA	NA	.01	.50	.30	2.5	0
77	1.3	15	388	24	.35	.10	.21	1.1	117
61	1.0	10	267	21	.35	.09	.19	1.0	92

FOOD	Water	Protein	Fat	Food Energy	Total Carbo-hydrates	Fibre	Calcium
per 100g edible portion	g	g	g	Calories	g	g	mg
Brussel Sprouts — raw	85	4.6	.5	49	8.7	1.6	32
— boiled	88	4.1	.5	38	6.6	1.6	30
Buckwheat — raw kernels	11	11.7	2.4	335	72.9	9.9	114
— flour	12	11.7	2.5	333	72.0	1.6	33
Bulghur Wheat	10	11.2	1.5	354	75.7	1.7	29
Butter — Salted	16	.8	81.3	727	.7	0	17
— Unsalted	16	.8	81.3	727	.7	0	17
Buttermilk	91	3.5	1.0	38	4.2	0	115
Butternut Squash — raw	88	1.4	.3	39	9.4	1.4	19
— baked	85	1.8	.4	50	11.7	1.8	24
— boiled	91	1.1	.3	30	6.9	1.4	17
Cabbage, Chinese — raw	95	1.4	.1	14	2.6	.6	46
Red — raw	90	2.0	.2	31	6.9	1.0	42
White — raw	92	1.5	.2	26	5.4	.8	47
— boiled	94	1.2	.2	22	4.3	.8	43
Canteloupes or Rockmelons	93	.7	.2	25	5.7	.3	17
Carob Powder — dry	11	4.5	1.5	180	80.7	7.7	352
Carrots — raw	89	.9	.2	36	8.6	1.0	40
— boiled	91	.8	.2	30	7.0	1.0	36
Cashew Nut kernels — raw	5	17.2	45.7	561	29.3	1.4	38
Cauliflower — raw	91	2.6	.2	26	4.6	1.0	21
— boiled	91	2.2	.2	24	4.2	1.0	20
Celery — raw	94	1.0	.1	18	3.9	.6	48
— boiled	95	.9	.1	17	3.1	.6	38
Cheese, Cheddar — natural	36	26.1	33.2	402	0	0	860
Cottage — creamed	78	13.6	4.2	106	2.9	0	94
— uncreamed	79	18.2	.4	91	2.4	0	93
Cream	54	9.0	32.0	345	3.4	0	40
Ricotta (50% whey)	79	16.7	1.8	100	2.5	0	NA
Swiss — natural	38	28.8	29.4	378	0	0	950
Cherries — raw	82	.9	.4	61	15.1	.3	18
Chestnuts — fresh, raw	53	2.9	1.5	194	42.1	1.1	27
— dried	8	6.7	4.1	377	78.6	2.5	52
Chicken — boiled	64	26.3	8.4	198	0	0	14
— fried	54	28.6	13.1	253	2.9	0	15
— roasted	60	29.1	9.4	199	0	0	16
Chickpeas(Garbanzos)—dry, raw	11	20.5	4.8	360	61.0	5.0	150
Chives — raw	91	1.8	.3	28	5.8	1.1	69
Chocolate — Plain dark	Tr	4.1	30.6	534	62.6	0	37
— Plain milk	Tr	8.9	31.0	538	56.4	0	295
Chayotes — raw	92	.6	Tr	28	7.0	.7	12
— boiled	93	.6	Tr	25	6.4	.7	11
Coconut — fresh meat	45	3.6	35.3	364	14.1	4.1	13
— dry meat shredded	4	6.8	63.0	672	29.0	4.0	23
— fresh milk (natural)	94	.3	.2	22	4.7	Tr	20
Cod Liver Oil	0	0	99.9	900	0	0	0

32

Phos-phorus	Iron	Sodium	Potassium	Magnes-ium	Vitamin A	Vitamin B1 Thiamine	Vitamin B2 Ribo-flavin	Vitamin B3 Niacin	Vitamin C Ascorbic Acid
mg	mg	mg	mg	mg	mg	mg	mg	mg	mg
79	1.3	13	420	29	.05	.10	.16	.7	97
71	1.0	10	300	21	.05	.08	.14	.6	83
282	3.1	NA	448	229	0	.60	.16	4.4	0
247	2.8	NA	NA	NA	0	.58	.15	2.9	0
338	3.7	NA	229	NA	0	.28	.14	4.5	0
16	.1	843	21	2	1.0	.02	.02	Tr	0
16	.1	8	15	2	1.0	.02	.02	Tr	0
96	.1	56	148	14	Tr	.04	.17	.1	1
31	.6	1	217	NA	.65	.05	.11	.6	11
39	.8	1	271	NA	.74	.05	.13	.7	10
26	.5	1	152	NA	.61	.04	.10	.4	6
40	.7	23	253	14	.01	.06	.08	.6	31
35	.8	26	268	NA	Tr	.09	.06	.4	61
30	.6	21	250	13	.01	.06	.05	.3	56·
21	.5	14	180	NA	.01	.04	.04	.3	42
16	.5	13	263	16	.34	.05	.04	.6	32
81	NA	NA	NA	NA	NA	NA	NA	NA	NA
36	.7	65	305	23	1.25	.06	.06	.6	6
31	.6	46	210	NA	1.17	.05	.06	.5	4
373	3.8	15	464	267	.01	.43	.25	1.8	0
64	.9	11	215	24	Tr	.08	.09	.5	52
58	.8	9	206	NA	Tr	.07	.08	.5	41
34	.5	135	332	22	.02	.04	.04	.4	7
29	.3	98	238	NA	.02	.03	.03	.3	5
506	.8	610	100	45	.42	.04	.48	.1	0
152	.3	229	85	NA	.05	.03	.25	.1	0
182	.3	290	72	NA	Tr	.02	.30	.1	0
140	.3	337	686	NA	.41	.02	.24	.1	0
NA	.1	NA	NA	NA	.03	.04	.16	.1	0
605	.9	157	100	NA	.37	.01	.40	.1	0
27	.4	2	192	14	.03	.05	.06	.4	8
88	1.7	6	454	41	0	.22	.22	.6	0
162	3.3	12	875	NA	0	.32	.38	1.2	0
265	1.9	98	381	19	.06	.05	.15	6.0	0
247	2.1	94	285	NA	.05	.07	.34	9.1	0
268	2.1	79	368	NA	.05	.08	.15	7.8	0
331	6.9	26	797	NA	.01	.31	.15	2.0	0
44	1.7	NA	250	32	.66	.08	.13	.5	56
287	NA	13	282	NA	.02	.09	.15	.6	0
242	1.8	125	413	58	.05	.12	.39	.6	0
NA	.5	20	NA	NA	Tr	.02	.04	.5	19
NA	.4	20	NA	NA	Tr	.01	.04	.4	14
95	2.0	19	480	46	0	.06	.02	.4	3
180	3.5	13	420	90	0	.04	.02	.5	0
13	.3	25	147	28	0	Tr	Tr	.1	2
0	2	0	10	0	29.47	NA	NA	NA	0

FOOD	Water	Protein	Fat	Food Energy	Total Carbo-hydrates	Fibre	Calcium
per 100g edible portion	g	g	g	Calories	g	g	mg
Corn (Maize) Meal – dry	12	9.2	3.9	355	73.7	1.6	20
Corn, Sweet – raw	73	3.6	1.2	97	21.0	.7	7
– boiled	77	3.2	1.0	83	10.8	.7	3
"Cornflakes"breakfast cereal–dry	3	8.6	.4	370	84.9	.7	5
Cream from Cows' Milk	57	2.1	38.0	364	3.0	0	82
Cucumbers – whole, raw	96	.6	.1	14	3.4	.6	26
– peeled, raw	96	.5	.1	13	3.1	.3	17
Currants, Black – raw	80	1.1	.1	59	15.0	2.8	49
Red – raw	84	1.2	.2	51	12.5	3.5	33
– dried	20	1.9	.5	273	72.8	NA	90
Dates, Californian–natural, dry	23	2.2	.5	274	72.9	2.3	59
Eggplant – raw	92	1.2	.2	25	5.5	.9	12
– boiled	94	1.0	.2	19	4.1	.9	11
Eggs (hen) – whole, raw	74	12.5	11.6	160	.7	0	54
– yolk, raw	50	16.2	30.6	347	.6	0	131
– white, raw	88	10.4	.2	49	.7	0	7
Figs – fresh, raw	79	1.3	.4	76	18.9	1.2	49
– dried	23	3.8	1.2	270	69.8	5.6	240
Flounder – baked	60	25.0	11.2	202	0	0	69
Flour – Rye (100%)	12	11.9	1.7	327	73.4	1.0	27
– Wheat, white self-raising	12	11.0	1.7	364	74.9	.4	93
fortified	12	11.0	1.7	364	74.9	.3	20
plain	13	11.0	1.7	360	73.9	.3	20
– Wheat, wholemeal	13	11.5	2.5	344	71.6	2.3	37
Garlic cloves – raw	61	6.2	.2	137	30.8	1.5	29
Gluten Flour – 45% wheat gluten	9	41.4	1.9	378	47.2	.4	40
Gooseberries – raw	87	.8	.3	43	10.7	1.9	20
Grapefruit – peeled, raw	89	.5	.2	37	9.2	.2	20
juice – fresh	89	.5	.1	36	8.5	.1	9
Grapes – raw	81	.7	.4	66	16.8	.6	18
juice – canned	83	.2	Tr	62	16.8	Tr	11
Guavas – fresh	82	1.0	.6	63	15.0	5.6	25
Ham – deboned, cooked	43	16.3	35.4	389	0	0	10
Haricot Beans – dry, raw	10	22.0	1.5	352	64.2	NA	146
– boiled	70	6.6	.4	120	24.0	NA	50
Hazelnut (Filbert)kernels –raw	6	12.6	62.4	634	16.7	3.0	209
Honey	19	.5	NA	322	80.0	0	6
Honeydew Melons – raw	90	.6	.3	34	8.1	.6	16
Kohlrabi – raw	91	2.1	.1	29	6.1	1.0	50
– boiled	92	1.8	.1	24	5.3	1.0	41
Lamb Chops (Chump) – medium broiled	50	18.6	30.7	355	0	0	10
Lard (and Dripping)	0	0	100.0	900	0	0	0

Phos-phorus	Iron	Sodium	Potassium	Magnes-ium	Vitamin A	Vitamin B1 Thiamine	Vitamin B2 Ribo-flavin	Vitamin B3 Niacin	Vitamin C Ascorbic Acid
mg	mg	mg	mg	mg	mg	mg	mg	mg	mg
256	2.4	1	284	NA	.06	.38	.11	2.0	0
115	.7	Tr	260	48	.04	.15	.12	1.7	12
89	.6	Tr	165	19	.04	.11	.10	1.3	7
57	8.8	990	200	16	.02	1.47	2.10	14.5	NA
60	.1	65	229	25	.50	.03	.12	.1	1
24	1.1	9	168	11	.03	.03	.04	.2	10
16	.3	9	168	NA	Tr	.03	.04	.2	10
34	1.2	3	360	15	.02	.04	.05	.3	209
29	1.0	2	234	15	Tr	.04	.03	.1	36
138	2.2	21	719	34	Tr	.14	.10	.5	3
63	3.0	1	648	58	Tr	.09	.10	2.2	0
26	.7	2	214	16	Tr	.05	.05	.6	5
21	.6	1	150	NA	Tr	.05	.04	.5	3
218	2.4	122	129	11	.28	.10	.30	.1	0
553	6.2	564	106	16	.76	.27	.41	Tr	0
15	.2	158	141	9	0	.02	.29	.1	0
28	.6	2	192	20	.01	.06	.05	.5	2
101	3.5	60	900	71	.01	.13	.12	1.7	0
244	1.4	237	587	NA	NA	.06	.08	2.5	2
269	2.7	1	203	NA	0	.30	.12	2.6	0
484	1.4	730	90	NA	0	.22	.05	1.3	0
87	2.9	2	90	25	0	.44	.26	3.5	0
87	1.4	2	90	25	0	.22	.05	1.3	0
372	3.2	3	370	113	0	.51	.09	4.1	0
202	1.5	19	529	36	Tr	.25	.08	.5	15
140	NA	2	60	NA	0	NA	NA	NA	0
35	.5	1	137	9	.03	.04	.02	.2	35
17	.3	1	187	12	Tr	.05	.02	.2	40
14	.3	1	147	12	Tr	.04	.02	.2	39
19	.5	2	194	13	.01	.05	.04	.2	4
11	.3	2	116	13	NA	.04	·.02	.2	Tr
35	.8	4	289	13	.03	.06	.04	1.2	251
192	2.4	1,106	201	NA	0	.63	.20	3.7	0
309	6.8	43	1,194	NA	.07	.44	.18	2.3	2
122	2.5	15	320	NA	.02	.08	.05	.6	0
337	3.4	2	704	184	NA	.46	NA	.9	Tr
9	.8	10	74	3	0	.03	.03	.3	1
16	.4	12	235	NA	Tr	.05	.03	.3	23
51	.6	9	382	37	Tr	.06	.05	.2	61
42	.5	7	278	NA	Tr	.06	.04	.2	43
165	2.0	91	410	17	NA	.11	.18	4.1	0
0	0	0	0	0	0	0	0	0	0

FOOD	Water	Protein	Fat	Food Energy	Total Carbo-hydrates	Fibre	Calcium
per 100g edible portion	g	g	g	Calories	g	g	mg
Leeks – raw	87	2.3	.4	43	9.1	1.1	56
– boiled	88	2.2	.3	38	8.0	1.1	54
Lemons – peeled, raw	90	1.0	.4	32	8.7	.4	31
juice – fresh	91	.4	.2	26	8.0	Tr	12
Lentils, Brown – dry, raw	10	24.1	1.1	336	61.7	4.0	58
– boiled	72	7.8	.3	110	20.3	1.3	20
Lettuce – raw	95	1.3	.3	17	3.0	.5	32
Lima Beans – dry, raw	12	20.6	1.4	339	62.2	4.3	69
– boiled	64	8.2	.7	130	24.6	1.7	28
Limes – peeled, raw	86	.8	.2	29	11.9	.6	40
juice – fresh	90	.3	.1	28	9.0	Tr	9
Linseed – whole, raw	6	18.0	34.0	498	37.2	8.8	271
Liver, Average all animals – raw	70	19.0	4.2	139	5.0	0	8
– floured and fried	46	29.4	10.5	269	14.0	0	10
Loganberries – raw	83	1.0	.6	60	14.4	3.0	35
Loquats – raw	84	.7	.2	56	14.4	.4	20
Lychees – raw	82	.9	.3	64	16.4	.3	8
Macadamia Nut kernels – raw	3	7.8	71.6	691	15.9	2.5	48
Mangoes – raw	82	.7	.2	66	17.2	.9	10
Maple Sugar – pure	8	Tr	Tr	348	90.0	0	143
Syrup – pure	33	Tr	Tr	252	65.0	0	104
Margarine – Cooking	15	.5	80.1	720	.8	0	18
– Table	15	.4	81.2	727	.6	0	20
Milk, Cows' – whole	88	3.3	3.8	67	4.6	0	115
Goats' – whole	88	3.2	4.0	67	4.6	0	129
Human – whole	87	1.2	3.9	69	7.4	0	31
Soya (average)							
– dry powder	5	34.1	11.9	423	40.1	2.0	330
– reconstituted	91	3.1	1.1	38	3.6	.8	30
Millet – whole grain	12	9.9	2.9	327	72.9	3.2	20
Miso (fermented soya beans & cereal)	53	10.5	4.6	171	23.5	2.3	68
Molasses – "Blackstrap"	24	NA	NA	213	55.0	NA	684
Mung Beans – dry, raw	11	24.2	1.3	340	60.3	4.4	118
– sprouted	89	3.8	.2	35	6.6	.7	19
Mushrooms – raw	91	2.2	.3	22	3.8	.7	7
Nectarines – raw	82	.6	.1	62	16.5	.4	4
Oats, Rolled – dry	9	13.8	7.8	388	69.9	1.2	55
– boiled	87	2.0	1.1	55	10.0	.2	8
Oils – Vegetable, refined	0	0	100.0	884	0	0	NA
Okras – raw	89	2.1	.3	34	7.5	1.0	87
– boiled	90	1.8	.3	32	7.2	1.0	80
Olives, Green – fresh	70	2.0	21.0	211	1.8	1.0	12

36

Phos-phorus	Iron	Sodium	Potassium	Magnes-ium	Vitamin A	Vitamin B1 Thiamine	Vitamin B2 Ribo-flavin	Vitamin B3 Niacin	Vitamin C Ascorbic Acid
mg	mg	mg	mg	mg	mg	mg	mg	mg	mg
53	1.1	7	330	23	.07	.11	.06	.5	18
50	1.0	6	320	NA	.06	.08	.05	.4	13
18	.7	2	135	NA	Tr	.05	.02	.2	47
12	.1	1	113	8	Tr	.04	.01	.1	37
334	7.2	33	757	80	.01	.46	.24	2.2	5
101	2.2	NA	240	NA	Tr	.09	.06	.6	0
28	.7	12	228	11	.30	.06	.08	.2	13
385	7.6	4	1,499	180	Tr	.48	.18	2.0	2
154	3.0	2	602	NA	0	.13	.06	.7	0
20	.6	1	100	NA	Tr	.04	Tr	.1	37
12	.2	1	104	NA	Tr	.02	Tr	.1	32
462	4.4	NA	NA	NA	0	.17	.16	1.4	0
336	10.4	87	288	15	8.4	.31	3.0	15.0	34
552	14.2	120	453	26	11.18	.27	3.8	15.7	28
20	1.3	1	170	25	.01	.03	.06	.3	26
36	.4	NA	348	NA	.07	NA	NA	NA	3
42	.4	3	170	NA	NA	NA	NA	NA	42
161	2.0	NA	264	NA	0	.34	.11	1.3	0
13	.3	7	189	18	.80	.06	.06	.9	41
11	1.4	14	242	Tr	NA	NA	Tr	Tr	0
8	1.2	10	176	Tr	NA	NA	Tr	Tr	0
NA	0	1,250	34	NA	.64	NA	0	NA	0
16	0	1,250	23	NA	.56	NA	0	NA	0
96	.1	56	150	13	.04	.04	.17	.1	1
106	.1	34	180	17	.04	.04	.11	.3	1
15	.1	14	51	4	.06	.01	.04	.2	4
680	9.0	500	1,640	250	.01	1.16	.33	2.2	0
62	.8	45	149	23	Tr	.11	.03	.2	0
311	6.8	NA	430	162	0	.73	.38	2.3	0
309	1.7	2,950	334	NA	Tr	.06	.10	.3	0
84	16.1	96	2,927	258	0	.11	.19	2.0	0
340	7.7	6	1,028	NA	.01	.38	.21	2.6	0
64	1.3	5	223	NA	Tr	.13	.13	.8	19
116	1.0	8	480	13	0	.01	.44	5.1	4
24	.5	4	307	13	.15	.07	NA	NA	19
371	4.1	4	354	144	NA	.58	.14	1.0	0
52	.6	NA	51	21	NA	.08	.02	.1	0
NA	NA	NA	NA	NA	NA	NA	NA	NA	NA
56	.7	2	235	41	.06	.13	.14	1.1	30
52	.6	2	200	NA	.06	.10	.11	.9	20
15	2.8	1	809	NA	.02	Tr	Tr	Tr	NA

FOOD	Water	Protein	Fat	Food Energy	Total Carbo-hydrates	Fibre	Calcium
per 100g edible portion	g	g	g	Calories	g	g	mg
Onions, young − raw	88	1.0	.2	45	10.5	.7	136
mature − raw	90	1.2	.2	35	8.2	.6	31
− boiled	92	1.0	.2	27	6.1	.6	27
Oranges − peeled, raw	86	.9	.3	45	11.1	.5	39
juice − fresh	88	.8	.3	43	10.6	.1	32
Oysters − raw	84	8.7	1.5	68	4.1	0	88
Parsley − raw	81	4.5	.8	55	10.0	1.8	260
Parsnips − raw	82	1.7	.5	70	16.4	2.0	54
− boiled	83	1.6	.5	65	15.3	2.0	50
Passionfruit − raw	75	2.5	.7	91	21.2	NA	13
Pasta, White − boiled	72	3.2	.4	114	23.2	.1	8
− dry	11	11.3	1.5	367	76.8	.3	24
Wholemeal − dry	13	11.5	2.5	344	71.6	2.3	37
Papayas — raw	88	.6	.1	41	10.5	.9	21
Peaches − raw	87	.6	.1	41	10.7	.6	7
− dried	21	3.2	.7	263	68.5	3.1	40
Peanuts − raw without skins	5	26.5	47.9	567	17.5	1.9	57
− roasted, with skins	2	26.4	47.6	580	21.3	2.8	73
Pears − raw	84	.4	.3	56	14.5	1.3	8
− dried	25	1.2	1.8	270	70.0	6.4	34
Peas, fresh − raw	78	6.3	.4	80	15.5	2.1	24
− boiled	81	5.4	.4	70	13.5	2.1	20
Pecan Nut kernels − raw	3	9.2	71.2	687	14.6	2.3	73
Pepitas (Pumpkin Seed kernels) − raw	4	29.0	46.7	553	15.0	1.9	51
Peppers, Mature Hot Red, whole − raw	74	3.7	2.3	93	18.1	9.0	29
Persimmons − raw	79	.8	.4	76	19.3	1.6	6
Pineapples − raw	85	.5	.2	52	13.5	.4	17
juice − canned	86	.4	.1	49	13.2	.1	14
Pignolia (Pinenut) kernels − raw	6	31.1	47.4	553	11.6	.9	NA
Pinon (Pinenut) kernels −raw	3	13.0	60.5	635	20.5	1.1	12
Pistachio Nut kernels − raw	5	19.3	53.7	594	19.0	1.9	131
Plums − raw	83	.7	.1	59	15.6	.4	15
Pomegranates− raw	82	.6	.3	66	17.1	.2	3
Pork Chops − "well done"	39	21.8	38.0	436	0	0	11
Potatoes − raw	80	2.1	.1	76	17.1	.5	7
− baked in skin	75	2.6	.1	93	21.1	.6	9
− boiled in skin	80	2.1	.1	76	17.1	.5	7
Prunes − fresh, raw	79	.8	.2	75	19.7	.4	12
− dried	28	2.1	.6	255	67.4	1.6	51
− canned	80	.4	.1	77	19.0	Tr	14
Pumpkins − raw	92	1.0	.1	26	6.5	1.1	21
− boiled	90	1.0	.3	33	6.9	1.1	23

Phos-phorus	Iron	Sodium	Potassium	Magnes-ium	Vitamin A	Vitamin B1 Thiamine	Vitamin B2 Ribo-flavin	Vitamin B3 Niacin	Vitamin C Ascorbic Acid
mg	mg	mg	mg	mg	mg	mg	mg	mg	mg
32	.9	5	228	NA	Tr	.05	.04	.4	25
40	.5	8	149	12	.01	.03	.04	.2	10
32	.4	6	103	NA	Tr	.03	.03	.2	7
22	.4	2	173	11	.03	.08	.03	.3	50
17	.3	2	163	11	.03	.08	.03	.3	49
149	5.7	73	121	24	.09	.15	.19	2.4	0
72	6.5	39	903	14	1.33	.13	.28	1.2	178
79	.7	12	541	32	Tr	.10	.11	.4	14
74	.6	11	505	NA	Tr	.07	.08	.3	9
59	1.3	28	348	29	Tr	Tr	.11	1.5	24
50	.4	1	57	18	0	.03	.01	.4	0
161	1.3	3	182	48	0	.12	.05	1.5	0
372	3.2	3	370	113	0	.51	.09	4.1	0
17	.3	3	234	NA	.13	.04	.04	.3	64
21	.5	2	195	10	.11	.02	.05	1.0	7
138	6.0	11	1,191	48	.21	.01	.20	5.3	16
400	2.4	4	700	206	Tr	.93	.17	17.4	Tr
404	2.7	4	720	175	Tr	.29	.17	16.9	Tr
11	.3	2	119	7	Tr	.02	.04	.1	4
48	1.1	7	573	31	Tr	.01	.18	.6	9
116	1.9	2	338	35	.08	.32	.16	2.6	26
100	1.8	1	216	NA	.07	.25	.14	2.0	20
289	2.4	Tr	603	142	.01	.86	.13	.9	2
1,144	11.2	NA	NA	NA	.01	.24	.19	2.4	0
78	1.2	NA	NA	NA	2.17	.22	.36	4.4	369
26	.3	6	242	8	.27	.05	.04	.1	14
9	.4	2	194	13	.05	.08	.03	.2	26
9	.5	1	142	NA	.01	.05	.02	.2	9
NA	NA	NA	NA	NA	Tr	.62	NA	NA	Tr
604	5.2	NA	NA	NA	Tr	1.28	.23	4.5	Tr
500	7.3	NA	972	158	.04	.67	NA	1.4	0
16	.4	1	223	9	.04	.05	.04	.5	4
8	.3	3	259	NA	Tr	.02	.02	.3	7
275	2.9	115	458	27	0	.73	.18	4.5	0
53	.6	3	407	22	Tr	.10	.04	1.7	20
65	.7	4	503	NA	Tr	.09	.04	1.5	16
53	.6	3	407	NA	Tr	.09	.03	1.2	16
18	.5	1	170	NA	.03	.03	.03	.5	4
79	3.9	8	694	40	.18	.09	.17	1.6	3
30	4.1	2	235	NA	Tr	.01	.01	.4	2
44	.8	1	340	12	.08	.05	.11	.6	9
26	.4	1	240	NA	.08	.03	.05	.6	5

FOOD	Water	Protein	Fat	Food Energy	Total Carbo-hydrates	Fibre	Calcium
per 100g edible portion	g	g	g	Calories	g	g	mg
Quinces – raw	84	.4	.2	57	15.0	1.7	11
Radishes – raw	95	1.0	.1	17	3.6	.7	30
Raisins – dried	20	1.5	.5	279	74.9	.9	68
Raspberries, Red – raw	84	1.1	.5	57	13.9	3.1	36
Rhubarb – raw	94	.6	.1	17	3.9	.7	101
Rice Bran – dry, raw	10	13.3	15.8	276	50.8	11.5	76
Polished – dry, raw	13	6.5	.6	357	81.0	.3	17
– boiled	73	2.0	.2	107	24.4	.1	7
Unpolished – dry, raw	12	6.9	2.0	359	78.4	.9	28
– boiled	70	2.3	.6	120	25.2	.3	11
Rutabagas – raw	89	1.1	.1	36	8.6	1.1	58
– boiled	90	.8	.1	34	8.0	i.1	55
Rye – whole grain	11	12.1	1.7	334	73.4	2.0	38
– flour (100%)	12	11.9	1.7	327	73.4	1.0	27
Safflower Seed kernels – raw	5	19.1	59.5	615	12.4	NA	NA
Sago – dry	12	.3	.2	358	90.8	NA	9
Salmon – baked	63	27.0	7.4	182	0	0	NA
Scallops – steamed	73	23.2	1.4	112	0	0	115
Semolina – dry	12	9.4	1.3	358	78.7	NA	18
Sesame Seeds – hulled, raw	5	18.2	53.4	582	17.6	2.4	110
– whole, raw	5	18.6	49.1	563	21.6	6.3	1,160
Shallot (eschalot) bulbs – raw	80	2.5	.1	72	16.8	.7	37
Soya Beans – fresh	69	10.9	5.1	134	13.2	1.4	67
– sprouted	86	6.2	1.4	46	5.3	.8	48
– dry, raw	10	34.1	17.7	403	33.5	4.9	226
– boiled	71	11.0	5.7	130	10.8	1.6	73
Soya Flour – "full fat"	8	38.6	21.9	419	24.3	2.3	205
Soya Grits – "low fat"	7	47.3	7.1	355	31.6	4.6	252
Spinach – raw	92	2.8	.3	25	4.1	.6	101
– boiled	91	2.5	.3	23	3.7	.6	92
Squash, Summer – raw	95	.8	.1	18	4.0	.6	22
– boiled	96	.7	.1	15	3.5	.6	21
Winter – raw	88	1.3	.3	45	10.4	1.4	20
– boiled	89	1.2	.3	40	9.0	1.4	20
Strawberries – raw	89	.7	.5	37	8.6	1.3	24
Sugar Cane crystals – raw	Tr	0	0	385	99.4	0	20
– brown	3	0	0	366	93.8	0	100
– refined	Tr	0	0	390	99.9	0	2
Sunflower Seed kernels – raw	5	24.0	47.3	560	19.9	3.8	120
Swiss Chard — raw	91	2.6	.4	30	5.3	.6	115
– boiled	90	2.6	.4	28	4.8	.6	105
Sweet Potatoes – raw	71	1.7	.4	114	26.3	.7	32
(yellow) – baked in skin	64	2.1	.5	141	32.5	.9	40
– boiled in skin	71	1.7	.4	114	26.3	.7	32

40

Phos-phorus	Iron	Sodium	Potassium	Magnes-ium	Vitamin A	Vitamin B1 Thiamine	Vitamin B2 Ribo-flavin	Vitamin B3 Niacin	Vitamin C Ascorbic Acid
mg	mg	mg	mg	mg	mg	mg	mg	mg	mg
18	.5	4	200	NA	Tr	.04	.03	.2	11
31	1.0	18	322	15	Tr	.03	.03	.3	26
130	2.2	49	840	33	Tr	.14	.09	.5	Tr
29	1.1	1	174	20	.01	.02	.07	.4	23
21	.5	8	282	16	.01	.02	.07	.2	10
1,386	19.4	Tr	1,495	NA	0	2.26	.25	29.8	0
111	.7	5	110	28	0	.08	.03	1.6	0
35	.2	NA	34	8	0	.03	.01	.4	0
282	1.7	9	214	88	0	.32	.05	4.6	0
90	.5	NA	70	29	0	.09	.02	1.4	0
39	.4	5	211	15	.05	.06	.07	1.0	36
39	.4	5	210	NA	.04	.05	.06	.8	27
376	3.7	1	467	115	0	.43	.22	1.6	0
269	2.7	1	203	NA	0	.30	.12	2.6	0
NA	NA	NA	NA	NA	NA	NA	NA	NA	0
29	.9	4	5	NA	NA	NA	NA	NA	0
414	1.2	116	443	NA	.03	.04	.16	7.3	0-
338	3.0	265	496	NA	0	NA	NA	NA	0
100	1.0	12	166	NA	0	.13	NA	2.0	0
592	2.4	NA	NA	NA	NA	.18	.13	5.4	0
616	10.5	60	725	181	Tr	.98	.24	5.4	0
60	1.2	12	334	NA	Tr	.06	.02	.2	8
225	2.8	NA	NA	NA	.08	.44	.16	1.4	29
67	1.0	NA	NA	NA	Tr	..23	.20	.8	13
554	8.4	5	1,677	265	Tr	1.10	.31	2.2	0
179	2.7	2	540	NA	Tr	.21	.09	.6	0
593	7.4	2	1,730	247	.01	.76	.29	2.1	0
634	9.3	Tr	1,942	NA	Tr	.87	.35	2.6	0
58	3.3	78	700	88	.94	.11	.20	.6	56
53	3.0	71	637	NA	.85	.10	.20	.5	33
22	.4	1	172	16	.03	.05	.09	.9	20
21	.4	1	141	16	.03	.04	.08	.7	11
33	.6	1	369	17	.48	.05	.12	.5	10
30	.5	1	360	17	.47	.04	.10	.4	6
26	.8	2	161	12	.01	.03	.06	.4	58
4	.2	8	70	Tr	0	0	0	0	0
20	1.0	38	350	Tr	0	0	0	0	0
0	.1	1	Tr	Tr	0	0	0	0	0
837	7.1	30	920	38	Tr	1.96	.23	5.4	0
NA	2.8	72	526	NA	.96	.06	.18	.4	30
NA	2.5	65	480	NA	.87	.05	.15	.4	18
47	.7	10	243	31	1.0	.10	.06	.6	21
58	.9	12	300	NA	.92	.09	.07	.7	17
47	.7	10	243	NA	.90	.09	.06	.6	10

FOOD	Water	Protein	Fat	Food Energy	Total Carbo-hydrates	Fibre	Calcium
per 100g edible portion	g	g	g	Calories	g	g	mg
Tangarines — peeled, raw	87	.8	.3	46	11.2	.5	37
Tapioca — dry	12	.5	.2	363	88.7	.1	10
Tomatoes — ripe, raw	94	1.1	.2	22	4.7	.6	15
— boiled	92	1.3	.2	26	5.5	.5	13
juice — canned	94	1.0	.2	20	4.1	NA	7
Tuna — canned in water	70	28.0	5.8	167	0	0	10
— canned in oil	53	25.6	19.5	288	0	0	7
Turnips — raw	93	.9	.2	29	6.4	.9	49
— boiled	93	.8	.2	28	6.2	.9	47
TVP (Textured Vegetable Protein) — hydrated (30% solids)	70	16.3	.3	NA	10.4	1.0	NA
Veal Chops — medium broiled	63	24.9	11.0	206	0	0	15
Vinegar, Apple Cider — filtered	94	Tr	0	14	5.9	0	6
Malt — distilled	95	NA	0	12	5.0	0	NA
Walnut kernels (light) — raw	4	14.8	63.7	648	14.9	1.7	84
Watercress — raw	93	2.2	.3	21	3.2	.7	192
Watermelons — raw	93	.5	.2	27	6.5	.3	7
Wheat, hard red — whole, raw	13	14.0	2.2	330	69.1	2.3	36
soft standard — whole, raw	14	10.2	2.0	326	72.1	2.3	42
soft standard — flaked & rolled	10	9.9	2.0	340	76.2	2.2	36
Bran — dry, raw	13	14.6	4.9	225	62.1	10.3	105
Germ — dry, raw	9	26.3	7.8	380	49.5	2.9	81
Whey — liquid	93	.9	.3	26	5.1	0	51
Powder — dry	5	12.9	1.1	349	73.5	0	646
Yams — raw	75	2.3	.2	96	22.6	.9	20
— boiled	75	2.2	.2	94	22.3	.9	19
Yeast, Brewers'	5	38.8	1.0	283	38.4	1.7	210
Torula	6	38.6	1.0	277	37.0	3.3	424
Bakers — compressed	71	11.3	.4	86	13.3	NA	21
— dry, active	5	40.9	1.8	303	41.5	NA	42
Yogurt, Cows' — skimmed milk	86	5.9	.1	55	6.9	0	140
— whole milk	84	4.4	3.6	78	5.7	0	147
Zucchinis — raw	95	1.2	.1	17	3.6	.6	28
— boiled	96	1.0	.1	12	2.5	.6	25

Phos-phorus	Iron	Sodium	Potassium	Magnes-ium	Vitamin A	Vitamin B1 Thiamine	Vitamin B2 Ribo-flavin	Vitamin B3 Niacin	Vitamin C Ascorbic Acid
mg	mg	mg	mg	mg	mg	mg	mg	mg	mg
20	.4	2	168	NA	.05	.07	.03	.2	31
20	.6	4	19	3	0	0	0	0	0
32	.6	4	287	14	.17	.07	.05	.8	24
27	.5	3	244	NA	.15	.06	.04	.7	23
18	.5	NA	244	10	.10	.05	.03	.8	17
290	1.6	875	275	NA	Tr	.05	.10	13.3	0
294	1.2	800	320	NA	.34	.04	.09	11.8	0
32	.5	48	245	20	0	.04	.07	.6	28
31	.5	47	240	NA	0	.03	.06	.5	17
NA	NA	NA	NA	NA	0	.11	.42	.7	0
267	3.7	214	214	18	0	.12	.28	7.1	0
9	.6	1	100	1	0	NA	NA	NA	0
NA	NA	1	15	1	0	NA	NA	NA	0
453	2.4	3	491	131	Tr	.39	.13	1.0	0
52	1.8	56	298	20	.49	.09	.16	.8	74
11	.3	1	105	NA	.06	.04	.04	.2	6
383	3.1	3	370	160	0	.57	.12	4.3	0
400	3.5	3	376	160	0	.43	.11	3.6	0
342	3.2	2	380	NA	0	.36	.12	4.1	0
1,223	13.5	11	1,050	490	0	.60	.30	21.7	0
990	9.9	5	1,020	336	0	2.20	1.3	9.5	0
53	.1	NA	NA	NA	Tr	.03	.14	.1	NA
589	1.4	NA	NA	130	Tr	.50	2.51	.8	NA
60	.6	NA	600	NA	0	.10	.04	.5	12
58	.6	NA	590	NA	0	.08	.04	.4	8
1,753	17.3	121	1,894	231	Tr	15.61	4.28	37.9	Tr
1,713	19.3	15	2,046	165	Tr	14.01	5.06	44.4	Tr
394	4.0	7	482	59	Tr	.55	1.73	16.4	Tr
1,291	20.5	52	1,998	NA	Tr	4.17	5.10	36.7	Tr
100	Tr	40	175	NA	0	.05	.20	.1	1
100	Tr	40	175	NA	.04	.05	.20	.1	1
29	.4	1	202	NA	Tr	.05	.09	1.0	19
25	.4	1	141	NA	Tr	.05	.08	.8	9

Guidance with Certain Foods

Many points of explanation and guidance must arise throughout the reading of so many food composition figures. It is hoped that most of these will be covered by the following notes. However if the reader is in doubt regarding any other items, it is suggested that this author's composite health book *From Soil To Psyche*, be read in conjunction with the present work, for it is only by an understanding of the holistic approach to health that a proper selection of dietary ingredients may be made.

Avocadoes

As the most popular and most prolific variety of avocado is the Fuerte (the green, smooth-skinned variety which ripens in America between late September and early December), the analyses for this fruit are given special mention. When compared with the nutrients contained in the average of all avocado varieties, it can be seen that the Fuerte is also the most nutritious and, consequently, the most flavorsome. Avocados are unique fruits in that they possess such high concentrations of natural fatty acids, potassium and magnesium. Their comparatively high cost is certainly justified by their high nutritional properties.

Beef

Of the many cuts of beef on the market, the most popular is the T-bone steak, guaranteeing its choice in this book. Unlike other cuts of meat herein listed, this is given two listings: one for when it is broiled very lightly, regarded as "rare"; the other when it is broiled heavily regarded as "well done". The reader will notice that the nutritional values for the latter are some 50% more than the former, but notice please that the water content of the "well done" steak is just a little over half that of the "rare," thereby accounting for much of the difference, but not all. Allowing for the significant reduction in water when steak is cooked well, one can simply deduce that there is also a reduction in nutritional values when considered in proportion to the water contents. It is thus clear that the heavy cooking of meat tends to reduce its nutritional value in much the same way as occurs with vegetables or any other food which is too heavily cooked. It will also be noted that beef, as with other meats, is not listed in its raw state — this would be of no more than academic value, as people rarely consume meat raw in this country.

Bread

The special comparisons among the seven varieties of bread make highly interesting reading. As a preliminary comment, it should be made known that this author has for years contended that bread is only a secondary food. However, it continues to form the staple of many diets and, for this reason, its nutritional properties must be investigated. The growing number of criticisms about white bread can now be seen to be amply justified. In terms of nutritional values, white bread rates lower than any other wheat bread in all but carbohydrates — and its value here is of little advantage when we note that the fibre component is so low. Rye breads are far more nutritious than white wheat bread in almost every nutrient. Yet white bread is often sold as "fortified" by added nutrients, thereby indicating how pitifully depleted it is in its standard state. Indeed, no breads rate well in nutrient content, with the exception of sodium, yet this is of no value to man as it is in the form of added common salt, itself a health inhibitor.

Bulghur Wheat

The most nutritious form in which to eat wheat is by sprouting it. The next is to have it cracked, steamed and dried — the product of this process being known as bulghur wheat. This is a Lebanese idea which is rapidly gaining popularity in the West due to its tastiness and nutritional superiority over wheat flour.

Buttermilk

This residue from butter-making contains many of the nutrients of the milk, with the notable exceptions of fat and vitamin A. Its very low fat content makes buttermilk a preferred drink to whole milk amongst a growing number of weight-conscious people (although fruit juices would be a far better drink for them).

Cabbage

An interesting comparison is offered between the three varieties submitted. Of these, it is obvious that Red is the most nutritious. The general advantage of cabbage in the diet, as with most green vegetables, is the significant offering of vitamin C and a basic general sprinkling of most other nutrients and food enzymes. These enzymes, as yet, are insufficiently tabulated for inclusion in analyses.

Carob

Unfortunately, too little research has yet been undertaken on this the oldest of nature's sweeteners. Originally called "St. John's Bread", carob was well known in biblical times and before. In more recent years, chocolate has become its substitute. Carob is a nutrient-rich natural food which grows as a bean, the pods of which are the edible portion, the seeds only for propagation. Its high carbohydrate value contains significantly more sugars than starches, reflected in the extraordinary level of sweetness for which carob is renowned. The pod also possesses a very high dietary fibre content. Carob is an excellent natural sweet food, free from the undesirable acids and drugs found in chocolate, such as oxalic acid, theobromine, caffeine, etc. Carob is considered to possess other nutritional properties, some of which have yet to be confirmed by specific analytical figures.

Cheeses

A far greater number of varieties of cheese are manufactured than the six listed in our tables. These were chosen as representatives because of their general popularity among health-conscious people. The inclusion of ricotta cheese is a first in such nutrient tables and reveals the important properties of this low-fat cheese. Note, also, that of all other cheeses, natural swiss has the lowest salt content, as revealed from the sodium table — it is also the highest in protein and calcium, two nutrients for which cheeses are often included in the diet. Healthiest cheeses are made from raw milk and have least chemical additives.

Coconut

Rarely is fresh coconut available in America's city markets. By the time whole coconuts travel from the tropical south, they are far from fresh, as indicated by their hardened, white meat. Fresh coconut meat is soft and jelly-like, obtained only from green coconuts in the tropics, the only location where the figures for fresh meat and fresh milk are properly applicable.

"Cornflakes"

Inclusion of this processed breakfast cereal was intended primarily to give a warning as to how one should guard against becoming too impressed by analyses of processed foods. "Cornflakes" is a coined word and should not induce the belief that the product is closely related to corn, as a comparison with corn meal will prove. When compared with other breakfast cereals, such as rolled oats and bulghur wheat, "cornflakes" rate lowest in most nutrients, except those nutrients in which artifically high levels have been achieved by the addition of synthetic chemicals — please refer to iron, sodium and the B vitamins. This practice is called "fortification" of nutrients and has become fairly standard practice in food processing when natural nutrients are diminished — particularly in fortified white wheat flour, margarine, processed breakfast cereals, etc.

Eggs

Egg white has no dietary advantages and can actually be constipating. An important consideration, not revealed by these tables, is that egg white represents almost pure protein, in the indigestible form of albumen — nearly 87% of its non-water component. The yolk is the really nutritive component of the egg, but its quantity in the diet should be determined by one's tolerance to cholesterol, of which egg yolk is exceptionally high. A significant improvement in the flavor of egg yolk is discernible from open-range, or free-range, eggs— those produced from fowls allowed to roam freely and not confined to battery production. Further flavor improvement will be noticed if the fowls are fed on organically-grown grains, etc. These flavor improvements indicate the increased mineral values in such egg yolks, especially in their lecithin content.

Figs, Dried

Figures shown are for the average of figs produced by the two major sources, Turkey and California. Note should be taken of the high fibre content of dried figs, as well as a good general balance of nutritional values. In general, these observations also apply to dates and other dried fruits, emphasising the fact that dried fruits offer the best source of "confectionary", especially for children.

Gluten Flour

Gluten is the protein of wheat, thereby offering special nutritional and baking properties, when prepared for use as gluten flour. However, such a high concentration of protein as in gluten is too much for the flour on its own, hence the addition of standard white wheat flour (55%) to 45% gluten to comprise the generally accepted mixture called gluten flour. The use of this should be carefully avoided by celiac sufferers — people suffering from a gluten intolerance.

Liver

Animal livers are highly regarded in some nutritional quarters as possessing ·valuable food properties. Certainly the nutrients revealed in the analysis tables substantiate such claims, except for calcium and magnesium. Liver is especially preferred for its iron and B-vitamin contents. However, it must be remembered that the liver of an animal is its major detoxifying organ and much of the animal's toxicity remains within the liver when it is prepared for human consumption. Does man really need this? Figures quoted are average for the livers of all animals used for human consumption.

Maple

When the sap flows in certain varieties of maple trees, it contains sweetness which has been prized for many centuries. The collected sap contains around 65% water, about half of which is evaporated in the "sugar house" near the plantation. The result is pure maple syrup. This is evaporated much further to produce maple sugar, thereby significantly concentrating the natural sugars. Care should be taken to avoid other than pure maple syrup or sugar, for many processors add "corn syrup" (little more than a cane sugar syrup) as an extender to reduce the high cost of pure maple. A special advantage of maple syrup is its *pH* rating (6.7 to 7.2), which is virtually neutral, thereby implying no risk of acidifying the saliva or damaging tooth enamel. Maple sugar, unlike cane sugar or honey, also possesses appreciable quantities of the minerals, iron, calcium and potassium.

Milks

When we compare the nutritional values of milk from cows and goats with that from the human breast, certain considerable divergencies become apparent. Human milk is much lower in protein, calcium and most other mineral elements, higher in carbohydrate (milk sugar in this case) and in vitamins A and C. Thus, if we are to accept that the Law of Creation knows what it is about, other milks are far less suitable to the needs of the human infant than its mother's milk, being too rich in some nutrients and too poor in others. Nutritional experience takes us even further than these analysed figures, proving to us in practice that infants fed on cows' milk often suffer acute or chronic pathological problems, the commonest of which are asthma, sinusitis and the many illnesses with which excessive mucus is associated. Of the two animal milks, goats' milk is certainly the more easily assimilated by the human infant, due to its simpler molecular structure and the fact that goats are, in general, far healthier animals than commercially-pastured cows. But even more easily digested, by infant and adult human alike, are soya bean milks or nut milks. Health food stores in most countries offer at least one readily-prepared soya milk, which is highly advantageous as this is not easily prepared in the home. Nut milks can be more easily prepared at home using peeled and ground almonds (buy them as naturals and prepare them yourself for best results) or cashew nut kernels.

Miso

Over recent years, ·the interest in the Japanese-originated macrobiotic diet has grown considerably throughout the Western world. One of the most highly-recommended foods in this diet is miso, thus it is included in these tables as representative of, and of guidance to, the increasing demand by young people for macrobiotics. Miso is a preparation made from specially-fermented soya beans and selected cereals. Sea salt is also added to the preparation, hence its high sodium figure. Few nutritionists recommend miso for general inclusion in the diet because of its fermentation and salt.

Pasta

This is the collective term used to describe all noodle-type preparations, the most common of which are spaghetti and macaroni. Such foods are generally regarded as being of Italian origin, although the long, slender noodle variety has been known to the Chinese for countless years. Wheat flour is the general basis for their manufacture, with an increasing demand for the use of wholemeal flour. Our tables show the comparison between the two in the dry state, highlighting the significant nutritional advantages of the wholemeal variety.

Rice

The complete nutrient tables afford an excellent comparison of the significant nutritional variation between unpolished and polished rice. When rice has its bran (polish) removed, its nutritional loss can be up to two-thirds, proving how important it is to always exercise your preference for unpolished (brown) rice. The fact that rice bran possesses such massive nutritional properties, yet is not especially palatable in itself, indicates how much more beneficial it is when intact, as part of natural, unpolished grain.

Sesame Seeds

Here we find another instance of superior nutritional qualities being available from the whole food. Unfortunately, in this case, the outer shell of the sesame seed is tough and bitter, hence the need to remove it. Alternatively, the whole seed can be ground into a meal, which will be quite dark, due to the color of the hull. However, a further problem with the hull is its content of calcium oxalate, a chemical compound which is an irritant to the kidneys and the bladder.

Soya Beans

One of nature's highest protein foods, the soya bean, is also one of the most difficult to prepare. Many people find cooked soya beans difficult to digest, resulting in the production of intestinal gas. This can be largely overcome by sprouting soya beans prior to cooking and by not combining with them, in the same meal, any concentrated carbohydrate food. There is some belief that soya beans possess certain enzymes which react adversely with human digestive enzymes, although this author has been unable to find conclusive proof of this claim. Two special dietary uses of soya beans are becoming more popular in these days of growing health-consciousness: Soya Grits and Soya Milk.

Soya Grits

Prepared from soya beans by being granulated, steamed, partially defatted and dried, soya grits offer a very palatable, nutrient-rich food. They can be eaten dry, used as a component of breakfast muesli, in vegetable casseroles, or as an alternative to granulated nuts in any suitable dish. Some people prefer them as a between-meal snack, but their high level of nutritional factors suggests that they are better eaten with meals, rather than between.

Soya Milk

Soya milk can be prepared at home from soya flour or by grinding one's own soya beans into a flour as required. However, neither method will provide results as palatable as when using one of the readily-prepared soya milks available from most health food stores. As a replacement for cows' milk, soya milk has manifold advantages, especially for infants — it is more easily assimilated, is not mucus-forming, does not have to be pasteurised and is, thus, far healthier. Soya milk contains no cholesterol (as do animal milks) and is richer in polyunsaturated fatty acids than saturated (animal milks are the reverse).

T.V.P.

This is registered trade name of the Archer Daniels Midland Company of Decatur, Illinois. This is an organisation which did much pioneering work in the development of Textured Vegetable Protein (or Soya Protein) as a meat substitute Composed, primarily, of soya bean flour, T.V.P. is the extruded product of meat-like flavor which some years ago swept the meat world with its almost undetectable similarity. It is flavored by vegetable and herb extracts, together with mineral salts, especially sodium chloride. By careful experimentation, these flavors have been developed to simulate beef, ham and chicken, etc. When prepared for eating, T.V.P. is reconstituted in hot water until it restores to a 70% water content, then cooked. It can be used by itself as a protein-rich main course food, or can be used in conjunction with a suitable meat as an "extender", such as many hamburger manufacturers now do. Advantageously, it is cholesterol-free and predominates in polyunsaturates.

Vinegars

Unfortunately, very little nutritional information is available for listing on the contents of malt vinegar. This is quite probably because very little nutrient value is obtained from it. Where direct comparisons are numerically available, it is obvious that apple cider vinegar has more nutrient value than malt, although even the former could not be regarded as nutrient-rich. Unfiltered, unpasteurised and undiluted apple cider vinegar, we would assume, has higher nutritional properties than the figures quoted, but such were not obtainable when this book went to print.

Yogurt

This milk product has risen sharply in popularity over recent years. And rightly so, for it affords a much easier means of assimilation for the human body than liquid milk can provide. Whether spelled as "yoghurt" or "yoghourt", or as listed here, no variation in the product is implied by different spellings — rather, do they follow national linguistic trends. The direct comparison between skimmed and whole milk yogurts should provide a valuable guide to their selection by consumers. For those seeking higher calcium or lower carbohydrate contents, the whole milk yogurt is most suited; for lower fat and calorie content, with higher protein values, skimmed milk yogurt will be preferred. Goats' milk yogurt provides an even more nutritious food, but the analyses of this were not completed when this book went to print. A further advantage of goats' milk yogurt is that its preparation is usually from raw unpasteurised milk. This implies that the animals producing such milk are extremely healthy, otherwise government regulations would insist that this milk be pasteurised.

Protein

Proteins are the most important nutrients sought by the human body through its food intake. They are also the most complex nutrients in terms of their chemical composition and formulation.

All foods contain some protein, whether they be of plant or animal origin. Protein of animal origin is chemically the more complex and more difficult for man to digest. It demands the consumption of larger quantities than would be needed of plant proteins for the same amount of usable protein to be made available to the human body.

Animal proteins in the human diet derive from meats, seafood, cheese, eggs, milk and poultry. They contain animal cholesterol and saturated fatty acids which can pose problems to the functioning of the human body if eaten in excess. Likewise, health problems can also be caused by the lack of dietary fiber in animal proteins unless the diet also includes reasonable amounts of vegetables and fruits. Animal proteins, nevertheless, are the most commonly consumed in Western countries, due to some skillful and misleading promotion. Many claims are made that animal proteins are more complete, provide humans with more strength and are less fattening than nuts or seeds. These claims are entirely false, as proven at length in this author's health book, *From Soil To Psyche*.*

Plant protein sources represent a far wider range of varieties, nutritional values and flavors. Dietetically, the most desirable for man are found in raw seeds and nuts, sprouted pulses (peas, beans and lentils) and grains. Plant foods provide man with the most easily digestible form of dietary protein, with nuts and seeds being the richest sources, as well as possessing all the essential amino acids. Nuts and seeds are far easier to store and prepare than meat, are also cheaper to produce and to purchase.

Quoted protein values of foodstuffs are actually assessments of crude protein and are determined by the quantitative methods. This uses as its basis the nitrogen content of the food, which is found by laboratory

From Soil To Psyche is published by Woodbridge Press, Santa Barbara, California.

analysis. The nitrogen value is then multiplied by factors varying from 5.18 to 6.38 to determine the quantity of total crude protein. These factors have been determined for each food, varying in accordance with the relationship between nitrogen and total protein. Nitrogen is an essential element in every amino acid molecule and it is the grouping of these amino acids which form food proteins.

The resultant number of grams of protein in each 100 grams of edible portion of food analysed is listed in the following graduated table. Thus, each figure for protein represents the percentage content of protein in each food. Following this table are extracts from the general Food Nutrient Tables for selected protein-rich foods. This allows direct comparisons of all other nutrients, as well as providing an important guide to protein-rich food selection.

PROTEIN

CONTENT RANGE IN EDIBLE FOODS — FROM THE HIGHEST DOWN
Measured in grams per 100 gram portion

Food	g	Food	g
Soya Grits — "low fat"	47.3	Bream fish — steamed	17.8
Gluten Flour	41.4	Cashew Nut kernels — raw	17.2
Yeast, Bakers' — dry, active	40.9	Cheese, Ricotta	16.7
Yeast, Brewers'	38.8	Ham — deboned, cooked	16.3
Yeast, Torula	38.6	T.V.P. — hydrated	16.3
Soya Flour — "full fat"	38.6	Eggs (hen) — yolk, raw	16.2
Soya Beans — dry, raw	34.1	Walnut kernels — raw	14.8
Soya Milk — dry	34.1	Wheat Bran — dry, raw	14.6
Beef Steak (T-bone)—"well done"	33.1	Brazil Nut kernels — raw	14.3
Pignolia (Pinenut) kernels — raw	31.1	Wheat, hard red, — raw, whole	14.0
Liver — floured & fried	29.4	Rolled Oats — dry	13.8
Chicken — roasted	29.1	Cheese, Cottage — creamed	13.6
Pepitas — raw, shelled	29.0	Rice Bran — dry, raw	13.3
Cheese, Swiss — natural	28.8	Pinon (Pinenut) kernels — raw	13.0
Chicken — fried	28.6	Whey Powder — dry	12.9
Tuna — canned in water	28.0	Hazelnut kernels — raw	12.6
Bacon — grilled	27.2	Eggs (hen) — whole, raw	12.5
Salmon — baked	27.0	Rye — whole grain	12.1
Peanuts — raw, without skins	26.5	Flour — Rye (100%)	11.9
Peanuts — roasted, with skins	26.4	Buckwheat — raw & flour	11.7
Wheat Germ — dry, raw	26.3	Flour — Wheat, wholemeal	11.5
Chicken — boiled	26.3	Pasta — Wholemeal, dry	11.5
Cheese, Cheddar — natural	26.1	Yeast, Bakers' — compressed	11.3
Tuna — canned in oil	25.6	Pasta, White — dry	11.3
Broadbeans — dried	25.1	Bulghur Wheat	11.2
Flounder — baked	25.0	Soya Beans — boiled	11.0
Veal Chops — medium **broiled**	24.9	Flour — Wheat, white	11.0
Mung Beans — dry, raw	24.2	Flour — Wheat, self-raising	11.0
Lentils, Brown — dry, raw	24.1	Flour — White, fortified	11.0
Sunflower Seed kernels — raw	24.0	Soya Beans — fresh	10.9
Scallops — steamed	23.2	Miso	10.5
Haricot Beans — dry, raw	22.0	Eggs (hen) — white, raw	10.4
Pork Chops — grilled	21.8	Wheat, soft — raw whole	10.2
Beef Steak (T-bone) — "rare"	21.5	Wheat, soft — flaked, rolled	9.9
Lima Beans — dry, raw	20.6	Millet — wholegrain	9.9
Chickpeas (Garbanzos)—dry, raw	20.5	Semolina — dry	9.4
Almond kernels — natural, raw	19.5	Pecan Nut kernels — raw	9.2
Pistachio Nut kernels — raw	19.3	Bread — Mixed Grain	9.2
Safflower Seed kernels — raw	19.1	Corn Meal — dry	9.2
Liver — raw	19.0	Cream Cheese	9.0
Sesame Seeds — whole, raw	18.6	Chocolate — Plain milk	8.9
Lamb Chops — medium **broiled**	18.6	Oysters — raw	8.7
Sesame Seeds — hulled, raw	18.2	"Cornflakes"breakfast cereal—dry	8.6
Cheese, Cottage — uncreamed	18.2	Bread — Cracked Wheat	8.5
Linseed — whole, raw	18.0	Broadbeans — raw, fresh	8.4

Continued next page

PROTEIN continued

Lima Beans — boiled	8.2
Bread — Wholemeal	8.1
Bread — Brown	8.0
Barley — pearled, dry	7.9
Bread — White	7.8
Lentils, Brown — boiled	7.8
Macadamia Nut kernels — raw	7.8
Bread — Dark Rye	7.6
Bread — Light Rye	7.6
Rice — Unpolished, raw	6.9
Coconut — dry meat shredded	6.8
Chestnuts — dried	6.7
Haricot Beans — boiled	6.6
Rice — Polished, raw	6.5
Peas, fresh — raw	6.3
Garlic Cloves — raw	6.2
Soya Beans — sprouted	6.2
Yogurt from skimmed Cows' Milk	5.9
Peas, fresh — boiled	5.4
Brussel Sprouts — raw	4.6
Apricots — dried	4.5
Carob Powder — dry	4.5
Parsley — raw	4.5
Bananas — dehydrated	4.4
Yogurt from Whole Cows' Milk	4.4
Brussel Sprouts — boiled	4.1
Chocolate — Plain dark	4.1
Figs — dried	3.8
Mung Beans — sprouted	3.8
Peppers, Mature Hot Red — raw	3.7
Broccoli — raw	3.6
Coconut — fresh meat	3.6
Corn, Sweet — raw	3.6
Buttermilk	3.5
Milk, Cows' — whole	3.3
Corn, Sweet — boiled	3.2

Milk, Goats' — whole	
Pasta, White — boiled	3..
Peaches — dried	3.2
Broccoli — boiled	3.1
Soya Milk — reconstituted	3.1
Artichokes, Globe — raw	2.9
Chestnuts — fresh, raw	2.9
Artichokes, Globe — boiled	2.8
Spinach — raw	2.8
Cauliflower — raw	2.6
Potatoes — baked in skin	2.6
Swiss Chard—raw or boiled	2.6
Passionfruit — raw	2.5
Shallot bulbs — raw	2.5
Spinach — boiled	2.5
Leeks — raw	2.3
Rice, Unpolished — boiled	2.3
Yams — raw	2.3
Avocadoes — Fuerte	2.2
Beet Greens — raw	2.2
Cauliflower — boiled	2.2
Dates, Calif. — natural, dry	2.2
Leeks — boiled	2.2
Mushrooms — raw	2.2
Watercress — raw	2.2
Yams — boiled	2.2
Asparagus — raw	2.1
Cream from Cows' Milk	2.1
Kohlrabi — raw	2.1
Okras — raw	2.1
Potatoes — raw or boiled	2.1
Prunes — dried	2.1
Sweet Potatoes (yellow) — baked	2.1
Cabbage, Red — raw	2.0
Oats, Rolled — boiled	2.0
Olives, Green — fresh	2.0
Rice, Polished — boiled	2.0

PROTEIN-RICH FOOD	Water	Protein	Fat	Food Energy	Total Carbo-hydrates	Fibre	Calcium
per 100g edible portion	g	g	g	Calories	g	g	mg
Almond kernels — natural, raw	5	19.5	53.8	598	18.9	2.6	245
Brazil kernels — raw	5	14.3	66.9	654	10.9	3.1	186
Cashew Nut kernels — raw	5	17.2	45.7	561	29.3	1.4	38
Hazelnut (Filbert) kernels — raw	6	12.6	62.4	634	16.7	3.0	209
Peanuts — raw, without skins	5	26.5	47.9	567	17.5	1.9	57
Pignolia (Pinenut) kernels — raw	6	31:1	47.4	553	11.6	.9	NA
Pinon (Pinenut) kernels — raw	3	13.0	60.5	365	20.5	1.1	12
Pistachio Nut kernels — raw	5	19.3	53.7	594	19.0	1.9	131
Walnut kernels (light) — raw	4	14.8	63.7	648	14.9	1.7	84
Pepitas (Pumpkin Seed) kernels — raw	4	29.0	46.7	553	15.0	1.9	51
Safflower Seed kernels — raw	5	19.1	59.5	615	12.4	NA	NA
Sesame Seeds — hulled, raw	5	18.2	53.4	582	17.6	2.4	110
Sunflower Seed kernels — raw	5	24.0	47.3	560	19.9	3.8	120
Soya Beans — boiled	71	11.0	5.7	130	10.8	1.6	73
TVP (Textured Vegetable Protein) — hydrated (30% solids)	70	16.3	.3	NA	10.4	1.0	NA
Eggs (hen) — whole, raw	74	12.5	11.6	160	.7	0	54
— yolk, raw	50	16.2	30.6	347	.7	0	131
— white, raw	88	10.4	.2	49	.7	0	7
Cheese, Cheddar — natural	36	26.1	33.2	402	0	0	860
Cottage — creamed	78	13.6	4.2	106	2.9	0	94
— uncreamed	79	18.2	.4	91	2.4	0	93
Cream	54	9.0	32.0	345	3.4	0	40
Ricotta (50% whey)	79	16.7	1.8	100	2.5	0	NA
Swiss — natural	38	28.8	29.4	378	0	0	950
Bacon — grilled	10	27.2	59.3	661	2.7	0	29
Beef Steak (T-bone) — "rare"	59	21.5	18.5	258	0	0	16
— "well done"	33	33.1	32.9	437	0	0	23
Chicken — boiled	64	26.3	8.4	198	0	0	14
Ham — deboned, cooked	43	16.3	35.4	389	0	0	10
Lamb Chops (Chump) — medium broiled	50	18.6	30.7	355	0	0	10
Liver, Average all animals — raw	70	19.0	4.2	139	5.0	0	8
— floured and fried	46	29.4	10.5	269	14.0	0	10
Pork Chops — broiled "well done"	39	21.8	38.0	436	0	0	11
Veal Chops — medium broiled	63	24.9	11.0	206	0	0	15
Bream fish — steamed	77	17.8	3.0	101	0	0	35
Flounder — baked	60	25.0	11.2	202	0	0	69
Oysters — raw	84	8.7	1.5	68	4.1	0	88
Salmon — baked	63	27.0	7.4	182	0	0	NA
Scallops — steamed	73	23.2	1.4	112	0	0	115
Tuna — canned in water	70	28.0	5.8	167	0	0	10
— canned in oil	53	25.6	19.5	288	0	0	7

N.B. Protein-rich foods are grouped for better comparison into vegetable and animal-origin types.

IN REPRESENTATIVE PROTEIN-RICH FOODS

Phosphorus	Iron	Sodium	Potassium	Magnesium	Vitamin A	Vitamin B1 Thiamine	Vitamin B2 Riboflavin	Vitamin B3 Niacin	Cholesterol
mg	mg	mg	mg	mg	mg	mg	mg	mg	mg
473	4.3	4	773	270	0	.24	.75	3.6	0
693	3.4	1	715	225	Tr	.96	.12	1.6	0
373	3.8	15	464	267	.01	.43	.25	1.8	0
337	3.4	2	704	184	NA	.46	NA	.9	0
400	2.4	4	700	206	Tr	.93	.17	17.4	0
NA	NA	NA	NA	NA	Tr	.62	NA	NA	0
604	5.2	NA	NA	NA	Tr	1.28	.23	4.5	0
500	7.3	NA	972	158	.04	.67	NA	1.4	0
453	2.4	3	491	131	Tr	.39	.13	1.0	0
1,144	11.2	NA	NA	NA	.01	.24	.19	2.4	0
NA	NA	NA	NA	NA	NA	NA	NA	NA	0
592	2.4	NA	NA	NA	NA	.18	.13	5.4	0
837	7.1	30	920	38	Tr	1.96	.23	5.4	0
179	2.7	2	540	NA	Tr	.21	.09	.6	0
NA	NA	NA	NA	NA	0	.11	.42	.7	0
218	2.4	122	129	11	.28	.10	.30	.1	550
553	6.2	564	106	16	.76	.27	.41	Tr	1,500
15	.2	158	141	9	0	.02	.29	.1	0
506	.8	610	100	45	.42	.04	.48	.1	100
152	.3	229	85	NA	.05	.03	.24	.1	15
182	.3	290	72	NA	Tr	.02	.30	.1	NA
140	.3	337	686	NA	.41	.02	.24	.1	120
NA	.1	NA	NA	NA	.03	.04	.16	.1	NA
605	.9	157	100	NA	.37	.01	.40	.1	85
292	2.7	3,328	462	25	0	.50	.31	5.1	NA
209	3.3	82	377	21	.01	.06	.16	4.3	70
322	5.0	126	580	NA	.02	.10	.25	6.7	105
265	1.9	98	381	19	.06	.05	.15	6.0	60
192	2.4	1,106	201	NA	0	.63	.20	3.7	70
165	2.0	91	410	17	NA	.11	.18	4.1	70
336	10.4	87	288	15	8.4	.31	3.0	15.0	300
552	14.2	120	453	26	11.18	.27	3.8	15.7	420
275	2.9	115	458	27	0	.73	.18	4.5	70
267	3.7	214	214	18	0	.12	.28	7.1	90
238	.6	113	281	NA	Tr	.06	.10	3.0	70
244	1.4	237	587	NA	NA	.06	.08	2.5	70
149	5.7	73	121	24	.09	.15	.19	2.4	250
414	1.2	116	443	NA	.03	.04	.16	7.3	70
338	3.0	265	496	NA	0	NA	NA	NA	NA
290	1.6	875	275	NA	Tr	.05	.10	13.3	70
294	1.2	800	320	NA	.34	.04	.09	11.8	70

N.B. As Vitamin C is nil in most of these foods, its space is better utilized by the figures for Cholesterol content, as shown in final column.

Fat

Fat is the common name used to embrace the major group of food nutrients found within the family of lipids. They all share the properties of being insoluble in water, yet digestible in the gastrointestinal tract of man. These fats are found in the cells of all living plants and their products, as well as in the fatty tissues of animals.

Digestible fats are essential nutrients in man's diet. They provide a convenient and easily assimilable form of food energy, as well as the construction of soft, fatty tissue within the body, so necessary for the protection of bones, organs and muscles.

The concentrations of fat in foodstuffs vary considerably, both in quantity and in chemical composition. Some are, obviously, more desirable than others in the diet — the most suitable being the polyunsaturated fatty acids. These are found primarily in plant foods, are easiest to digest and thus generally induce the least accumulation of fat in the body. Next, in terms of ease of digestion and assimilation, come the mono-unsat-urated fatty acids. Last are the saturated fatty acids.

Heading the list of fat content of foods are two with 100% fats: refined vegetable oils and lard (or "drip-ping"). These two items, therefore, possess no other nutrients of any consequence, containing only fatty acids. Lard is the fat of animals and, as such, contains a high proportion of saturated fatty acids, causing it to be solid at room temperatures. By contrast, vegetable oils are composed of a majority of unsaturated fatty acids, except in the case of coconut oil — its high concentra-tion of saturated fatty acids causing it to also become solid at room temperatures.

The commercial extraction and refining of vegetable oils, effectively removes all nutrients with the exception of a few traces of occasional vitamins, minerals and carbohydrates. When oils are extracted by the cold-press method (expeller extraction, free from the influ-ence of chemical solvents), somewhat more vitamins and minerals are retained. This is especially apparent if the oils remain unrefined.

Fat concentration in edible foods has been divided into two graduated tables. The first lists foods from the richest down to 1.8% fat content. Many of the foods in this list are shown with a more detailed analysis of their fat contents on pages 46 and 47. The second is a reverse list of foods with graduated concentrations from the lowest fat content to 1%. This will be especially helpful to people on a low-fat diet.

All foods have their fat contents measured as grams per 100 grams of edible portion, that is as a weight percentage.

FAT (1)

CONTENT RANGE IN EDIBLE FOODS – FROM THE HIGHEST DOWN

Measured in grams per 100 gram portion

Oils – vegetable, refined	100.0	Rice Bran – dry, raw	15.8
Lard (and dripping)	100.0	Chicken – fried	13.1
Cod Liver Oil	99.9	Soya Milk – dry	11.9
Butter – unsalted	81.3	Eggs (hen) – whole, raw	11.6
Butter – salted	81.3	Flounder – baked	11.2
Margarine – Table	81.2	Veal Chops – medium broiled	11.0
Margarine – Cooking	80.1	Liver – floured & fried	10.5
Macadamia Nut kernels – raw	71.6	Chicken – roasted	9.4
Pecan Nut kernels – raw	71.2	Chicken – boiled	8.4
Brazil Nut kernels – raw	66.9	Wheat Germ – dry, raw	7.8
Walnut kernels – raw	63.7	Rolled Oats – dry	7.8
Coconut – dry meat shredded	63.0	Salmon – baked	7.4
Hazelnut kernels – raw	62.4	Soya Grits – "low fat"	7.1
Pinon (Pinenut) kernels – raw	60.5	Tuna – Canned in water	5.8
Safflower Seed kernels – raw	59.5	Soya Beans – boiled	5.7
Bacon – grilled	59.3	Soya Beans – fresh	5.1
Almond kernels – natural, raw	53.8	Wheat Bran – dry, raw	4.9
Pistachio Nut kernels – raw	53.7	Chickpeas (Garbanzos) – dry, raw	4.8
Sesame Seeds – hulled, raw	53.4	Miso	4.6
Sesame Seeds – whole, raw	49.1	Cheese, Cottage – creamed	4.2
Peanuts – raw, without skins	47.9	Liver – raw	4.2
Peanuts – roasted, with skins	47.6	Chestnuts – dried	4.1
Pignolia (Pinenut) kernels – raw	47.4	Goats' Milk, whole	4.0
Sunflower Seed kernels – raw	47.3	Corn Meal – dry	3.9
Pepitas – raw, shelled	46.7	Human Milk, whole	3.9
Cashew Nut kernels – raw	45.7	Cows' Milk, whole	3.8
Cream from Cows' Milk	38.0	Yogurt from whole Cows' Milk	3.6
Pork Chops – broiled	38.0	Bream fish – steamed	3.0
Ham – deboned, cooked	35.4	Millet – while grain	2.9
Coconut – fresh meat	35.3	Bread – Mixed Grain	2.8
Linseed – whole, raw	34.0	Bread – Cracked Wheat	2.5
Cheese, Cheddar – natural	33.2	Flour – Wheat, wholemeal	2.5
Beef Steak (T-bone)–"well done"	32.9	Pasta, Wholemeal – dry	2.5
Cream Cheese	32.0	Buckwheat flour	2.5
Chocolate – Plain milk	31.0	Buckwheat – raw kernels	2.4
Lamb Chops – medium broiled	30.7	Bread – Wholemeal	2.4
Eggs (hen) – yolk, raw	30.6	Peppers, Mature Hot Red – raw	2.3
Chocolate – plain dark	30.6	Wheat, hard red – whole, raw	2.2
Cheese, Swiss – natural	29.4	Rice – Unpolished, raw	2.0
Soya Flour – "full fat"	21.9	Wheat, soft – whole, raw	2.0
Olives, Green – fresh	21.0	Wheat, soft – flaked & rolled	2.0
Tuna – canned in oil	19.5	Gluten Flour	1.9
Beef Steak (T-bone) – "rare"	18.5	Bread – Brown	1.8
Soya Beans – dry, raw	17.7	Cheese, Ricotta	1.8
Avocadoes – "Fuerte" variety	17.0	Pears – dried	1.8
Avocadoes – Av. all varieties	15.8	Yeast, Bakers' – dry, active	1.8

CONTENT RANGE IN EDIBLE FOODS – FROM THE LOWEST UP

Measured in grams per 100 gram portion

Sugar Cane crystals – all	0	Coconut – fresh milk	.2
Vinegar – cider or malt	0	Currants, Red – raw	.2
Apple juice – canned	Tr	Egg plant – raw or boiled	.2
Chayotes – raw or boiled	Tr	Eggs (hen) – White, raw	.2
Grape juice – canned	Tr	Garlic cloves – raw	.2
Maple Syrup – pure	Tr	Grapefruit – peeled, raw	.2
Maple Sugar – pure	Tr	Lemon juice – fresh	.2
Marrows (vegetable) – raw	Tr	Limes – raw	.2
Apricot nectar – canned	.1	Loquats – raw	.2
Artichokes, Jerusalem – raw	.1	Mangoes – raw	.2
Beets – raw or boiled	.1	Mung Beans – sprouted	.2
Cabbage, Chinese – raw	.1	Onions (all) – raw or boiled	.2
Celery – raw or boiled	.1	Pineapples – raw	.2
Cucumbers – whole or peeled	.1	Prunes – fresh, raw	.2
Currants, Black – raw	.1	Quinces – raw	.2
Grapefruit juice – fresh	.1	Rice – Polished, boiled	.2
Kohlrabi – raw or boiled	.1	Sago – dry	.2
Lime juice – fresh	.1	Tapioca – dry	.2
Nectarines – raw	.1	Tomatoes – raw, boiled or juice	.2
Papayas — raw	.1	Turnips – raw or boiled	.2
Peaches – raw	.1	Watermelons – raw	.2
Pineapple juice – canned	.1	Yams – raw or boiled	.2
Plums – raw	.1	Apples – peeled, raw	.3
Potatoes – raw, baked or boiled	.1	Bananas – ripe, raw	.3
Prune juice	.1	Beet Greens – raw	.3
Pumpkin – raw	.1	Breadfruit – raw	.3
Radish – raw	.1	Broccoli – raw or boiled	.3
Rhubarb – raw	.1	Butternut Squash – raw or boiled	.3
Rutabagas – raw or boiled	.1	Chives – raw	.3
Shallot bulbs – raw	.1	Gooseberries – raw	.3
Squash, Summer – raw or boiled	.1	Honeydew Melons – raw	.3
Yogurt from Skimmed Cows' Milk	.1	Leaks – boiled	.3
Zucchini – raw or boiled	.1	Lentils – boiled	.3
Apricots – raw	.2	Lettuce – raw	.3
Artichokes, Globe – raw or boiled	.2	Lychees – raw	.3
Asparagus – raw or boiled	.2	Mushrooms – raw	.3
Beans (long green) – raw or boiled	.2	Okras – raw or boiled	.3
Beet Greens – boiled	.2	Oranges – fruit and juice	.3
Bell Peppers — raw	.2	Pears – raw	.3
		Pomegranates – raw	.3
Cabbage, Red – raw	.2	Pumpkins – boiled	.3
Cabbage, White – raw or boiled	.2	Spinach – raw or boiled	.3
Canteloupe – raw	.2	Squash, Winter – raw or boiled	.3
Carrots – raw or boiled	.2	T.V.P. – hydrated	.3
Cauliflower – raw or boiled	.2	Tangarines — peeled, raw	.3

Continued next page

FAT (2) continued

		Dates, Calif. — natural, dry	.5
		Parsnips — raw or boiled	.5
Watercress — raw	.3	Raisins — dried	.5
Whey — liquid	.3	Raspberries, Red — raw	.5
Apples — dried	.4	Strawberries — raw	.5
Broadbeans — fresh, raw	.4	Sweet Potatoes (yellow) — baked	.5
Butternut Pumpkins — boiled	.4	Apples — with peel, raw	.6
Cheese, Cottage — uncreamed	.4	Cherimoyas — raw	.6
Cherries — raw	.4	Guavas — fresh	.6
"Cornflakes" — dry	.4	Loganberries — raw	.6
Figs — fresh, raw	.4	Prunes — dried	.6
Grapes — raw	.4	Rice, Polished — dry, raw	.6
Haricot Beans — boiled	.4	Rice, Unpolished — boiled	.6
Leeks — raw	.4	Lima Beans — boiled	.7
Pasta, White — boiled	.4	Passionfruit — raw	.7
Peas, fresh — raw or boiled	.4	Peaches — dried	.7
Persimmons — raw	.4	Bananas — dehydrated	.8
Sweet Potatoes — raw or boiled	.4	Parsley — raw	.8
Swiss Chard — raw or boiled	.4	Blackberries — raw	1.0
Yeast, Bakers' — compressed	.4	Corn, Sweet — boiled	1.0
Brussel Sprouts — raw or boiled	.5	Yeast, Brewers'	1.0
Currants — dried	.5	Yeast, Torula	1.0

Fatty Acids
and Cholesterol

As a guide to the fatty acid and cholesterol compositions of edible foods with high fat concentrations, the following table will be of great value. People with existing health problems related to fat or cholesterol in their diets will find this table especially helpful in assisting them to more wisely prepare their meals.

It is important to note that cholesterol in the diet comes only from foods of animal origin. Cholesterol, although a lipid, is not a fatty acid. Chemically, it is classed as a sterol, but it is associated with fats in the bloodstream of mammals, where it is used to transport fats to those parts of the body most needing them. Natural cholesterol forms compounds with the fatty acids as an expedient means of supplying fuel to the muscles for energy and also for the positioning of fats around the body for the building up of fatty tissue.

Adequate natural cholesterol is synthesised by man and all other mammals within their own bodies from their basic food requirements. Thus, when man consumes the flesh, blood, milk or organs of another animal, he ingests foreign cholesterol.

The inclusion of foreign cholesterol in the diet of any primate creates problems. As the highest of the primates and the only one which attempts carnivorism, man is the only animal to suffer from the effects of foreign cholesterol in the body. This comes about because the body prefers to use its own adequate natural cholesterol for its purposes and has no use for foreign cholesterol.

Finding no employment in the bodily activities, foreign cholesterol consumed by man will accumulate in his body, invariably being shunted out of the way like an unwanted child. A favorite resort of this cholesterol is behind the arterial valves where, in small quantities, it can be hidden to prevent impeding the work of natural cholesterol. Unfortunately, small quantities have the habit of accumulating — a build-up in foreign cholesterol eventually blocking the opening of arterial valves thereby stopping blood flow through the artery. Obviously, this can lead to a variety of pathological problems.

Most health practitioners are now advising patients to minimise their intake of cholesterol-containing foods, giving rise to the importance of the following table. In fact, the ideal human diet is composed of foods devoid of animal cholesterol, deriving nourishment only from vegetable foods. However the huge investment and prestige of the meat and dairy industries, and their influence in the diet field, currently propagate against the universal recognition of man's vegetarian heritage.

Although the figures for cholesterol in foods in the following table appear only for nineteen items, they are a vital guide to each type of food represented. For instance, most fish and animal flesh foods have a cholesterol content of 70 mg per 100 g edible portion. Eggs, organ meats and shellfish are significantly above this level. All measurements for cholesterol are tabulated as milligrams per 100 grams edible portion.

Let us now look to the fatty acid content of selected foods. From the analyses for total fat content have been selected the three basic types of fatty acid compounds in foods. Total saturated fatty acids are all grouped together in the second column. Oleic acid, being the most prolific mono-unsaturated fatty acid, occupies the third column. Linoleic acid, as the most representative of the polyunsaturated fatty acids, appears in the fourth column.

Saturated fatty acids are chemically the most complex. Due to the saturation of their electron structure, they do not easily combine with other nutrient compounds or mineral elements, thereby being the most difficult for the body to appropriate. Fortunately, they are only found in small quantities in plant foods, although they are much more prolific in foods of animal origin. These fats have the physical appearance of being solid at room temperatures, such as we see in butter, lard, etc.

Mono-unsaturated fatty acids have an ability to combine with one other element or compound, allowing more ease of digestibility than saturated fatty acids, yet

not the degree of flexibility offered by the polyunsaturates. Mono-unsaturated fatty acids are found to be
most abundant in olives and in nuts, while polyunsaturated fatty acids are most abundant in seeds.

Polyunsaturated fatty acids might be regarded as the
polygamists of the fatty acid family. They possess the
ability of combining with two or more elements or
chemical compounds and constitute the largest group
of fatty acids in the botanical kingdom. Regarded as the
most easily digestible, three acids within this group are
essential to body growth and energy supply. Of these,
linoleic (linolenic and arachidonic are the other two) is
especially important for its ability to combine with and
reduce foreign cholesterol in the body. As will be seen
in the following table, linoleic acid is most abundant in
safflower oil (72%), making it the most desirable oil for
those who insist on including animal foods in their diet.
(See page 48.)

All measurements of fatty acids are made in grams
per 100 gram edible portion of food, thereby giving a
direct percentage figure for each.

TABLE OF FATTY ACIDS AND CHOLESTEROL IN SELECTED FOODS

Food	Total Fat	Total Saturated Fatty Acids	Oleic Acid (Mono-unsaturated)	Linoleic Acid (Polyunsat.)	Cholesterol
per 100g edible portion	g	g	g	g	mg
Almond kernels – natural, raw	53.8	4	36	11	0
Avocadoes – Average all varieties	15.8	3	7	2	0
– Fuerte variety	17.0	3	8	2	0
Bacon – grilled	59.3	19	29	6	NA
Beef Steak (T-bone) – "rare"	18.5	9	8	Tr	70
Brazil Nut kernels – raw	66.9	13	32	17	0
Butter	81.3	46	27	2	250
Buttermilk	1.0	Tr	Tr	Tr	NA
Cashew Nut kernels – raw	45.7	8	32	3	0
Cheese, Cheddar – natural	33.2	18	11	1	100
Cheese, Cottage – creamed	4.2	2	1	Tr	15
Cheese, Cream	32.0	18	10	1	120
Cheese, Swiss – natural	29.4	16	9	1	85
Chicken – fried	13.1	3	7	2	60
Chickpeas (Garbanzos) – dry, raw	4.8	Tr	2	2	0
Coconut – fresh meat	35.3	30	2	Tr	0
– dry meat shredded	63.0	54	5	Tr	0
Cream from Cows' milk	38.0	21	12	1	0
Eggs (hen) – whole, raw	11.6	4	5	1	550
– yolk, raw	30.6	10	13	2	1,500
Hazelnut kernels – raw	62.4	3	34	10	0
Lamb Chops – medium broiled	30.7	17	11	1	70
Lard (and dripping)	100.0	38	46	10	95
Liver – Average all animals, raw	4.2	2	2	Tr	300
Margarine – hydrogenated	81.0	18	47	14	NA
– using liquid oil	81.0	19	31	29	NA
Milk – Cows', whole	3.8	2	1	Tr	11
– Goats', whole	4.0	2	1	Tr	NA
– Human, whole	3.9	2	1	Tr	NA
– Soya ("Soyvita"), dry	11.9	2	3	6	0
Millet – whole grain	2.9	1	1	1	0
Miso (fermented Soybeans & cereal)	4.6	1	1	2	0
Oats, Rolled – dry	7.8	2	3	3	0
Oils, refined – Corn	100.0	10	28	53	0
– Cottonseed	100.0	25	21	50	0
– Olive	100.0	11	76	7	0
– Peanut	100.0	18	47	29	0
– Safflower	100.0	8	15	72	0
– Sesame	100.0	14	38	42	0
– Soy	100.0	15	20	52	0
– Sunflower	100.0	12	20	63	0

Continued next page

Food	Total Fat	Total Saturated Fatty Acids	Oleic Acid (Mono-unsaturated)	Linoleic Acid (Polyunsat.)	Cholesterol
per 100g edible portion	g	g	g	g	mg
Olives, Green – fresh	21.0	2	16	2	0
Oysters – raw	1.5	1	Tr	Tr	250
Peanuts – raw, with skins	47.5	10	20	14	0
Pecan Nut kernels – raw	71.2	5	45	14	0
Pepitas – raw shelled	46.7	8	17	20	0
Pistachio Nut kernels – raw	53.7	3	35	10	0
Pork Chops – broiled	38.0	14	16	3	70
Safflower Seed kernels – raw	59.5	5	9	43	0
Salmon – baked	7.4	4	2	Tr	70
Sesame Seeds – whole, raw	49.1	7	19	21	0
– hulled, raw	53.4	7	20	22	0
Soya Beans – fresh or boiled	5.1	1	1	3	0
– dry, raw	17.7	3	4	9	0
Soya Flour – "full fat"	21.9	3	4	12	0
Sunflower Seed kernels – raw	47.3	6	9	30	0
Tuna – canned in oil	19.5	5	4	7	70
Veal Chops – medium broiled	11.0	6	5	Tr	90
Walnut kernels – raw	63.7	4	10	40	0
Wheat Germ – dry, raw	7.8	1	2	4	0
Yogurt from Whole Cows' Milk	3.6	2	1	Tr	11

77

Edible Oils

Although occupying a relatively small proportion of the human diet, edible oils are subject to some of the most conflicting and divergent opinions. Unfortunately, most people who express such opinions have not undertaken sufficient study or research to be scientifically correct in their utterances.

Extraction

Oil-bearing sources, such as seeds, beans or grains, are first crushed, then fed into an expeller extractor. This squeezes out some 30% of the available oil. It is this oil which is described at "expeller extracted" or, as is more commonly termed, "cold pressed". Actually, a certain amount of heat is generated by internal friction as the oil is being expelled and it is true that this heat would destroy some of the vitamins B_1 and C. However, oils contain such a low content of these vitamins that no real loss occurs. At least the buyer of cold-pressed oils is assured of a chemical-free product, the only further processing to which some oils are subjected is filtering, a form of refining which separates the oil from any residues of the source material.

The residue of expeller extraction is a mash which still contains some 70% of potential oil. Commercial processors recover this oil by dissolving the mash in a chemical solvent (usually hexane). The solvent is then evaporated, although we can never be guaranteed that all the solvent is removed from the oil. Further chemicals are then used in deodorizing, anti-oxidizing, winterizing, etc, as is deemed necessary to give this oil an increased shelf-life and buyer acceptability. By contrast, unrefined cold-pressed oils retain their natural wholesomeness in the form of vitamin-rich anti-oxidants. Unrefined oils, therefore, are the first choice of health-conscious people, whenever such oils are available.

Bottling

In spite of proven evidence to the contrary, some bottlers of edible oils persist in claiming that oils must be stored in dark bottles to "avoid deterioration". Indeed, oils should always be protected from direct sunlight and heat, but indirect light has no effect whatsoever on any properties of edible oils. No research appears to have yet been carried out on whether ultraviolet light has any affect on edible oils. However, if ultraviolet light were found to have any detrimental affect, it would not matter what color bottles were used to store oils, as all glass is a known filter of ultraviolet radiation. A disadvantage of dark bottles or cans is that they deprive the prospective buyer from observing the color and density of the oil.

Processing

The use of edible oils in food manufacturing is a significant cause of their loss of nutritional properties. In particular, the hydrogenation converts any polyunsaturated oils into saturated fatty acids; this especially taking place in the manufacturing of some margarines and many types of commercial mayonnaises.

A more serious danger attends the subjecting of edible oils to the high temperatures of cooking. This will induce varying degrees of molecular restructuring of the fatty acids which, in common terms, means that they will tend to become carcinogenic (cancer causing). This is especially likely when heated oils are reused, such as is usually done in restaurants and "fast food" establishments. If one proposes cooking with oil, it is wise to select an oil with a high boiling point, such as sesame, sunflower, safflower or soy and to insist on an oil which has retained most of its natural body, obviously a cold-pressed oil, desirably unrefined.

Food Energy—
Calories

The term "calorie", as used to denote the energy content of foods, is somewhat misleading. In actual practice, the unit used to measure the energy potential of foods is the Kilogram Calorie, abbreviated to Kcal. However, the convenience of modern usage has contracted this term to "calorie."

In 1968 a universal recommendation was made to use the term "joule" as the standard unit of energy content of foods. Although the joule is the more convenient, modern usage has virtually ignored the recommended change and persisted with "calorie" as indicating the food energy content. This book has bowed to modern usage for the convenience of readers, although those who prefer the more scientifically correct term may convert "calories" to "joules" by use of the conversion factor of 1 kilocalorie = 4.186 kilojoules.

Determination of the energy potential of foods has taken into account losses occurring during the food's metabolism within the body. Therefore, the figures quoted for a food's calorie content refer only to the net food energy available after the food has been thoroughly digested.

It is well known that when available food energy (measured in "calories"), is not utilized by the body, it is usually stored within that body in anticipation of a future need. This storage is in the form of bodily fat. Thus have people come to relate a food's calorie content with the accumulation of excessive fatty tissue around the body. This is often a valid relationship, implying that either less food or more exercise are required, or both. But it does not necessarily follow that all foods high in calories are fattening. Other nutritional factors, together with the food's general digestive properties, must be taken into account.

For example, many people attribute to nuts and to seeds the reputation of being fattening. This is a valid claim only when nuts and seeds are roasted and salted and/or when they are eaten as snacks between meals. But when raw nuts or seeds are eaten in suggested quantities with meals, they provide important sources of protein and are certainly not fat-producing. Quantities of up to four or five ounces of nuts per day, or up to three ounces of seeds per day, with fresh vegetables or fruits, will provide the average person's basic daily protein requirements and offer a delicious meal from which all nutrients (including calories) will be utilized.*

To allay fears of foods causing weight problems, it is far better for the person to consult a trained nutritionist than to be guided merely by a food's calorie content. Many natural foods are high in calories, but their valuable nutritional properties imply that they should be regarded as vital components of man's ideal diet.

As a convenient guide to the calorie content of foods, two sets of tables are offered. The first contains those foods with the highest calorie contents, graduated from the richest down to 100 calories. The second graduated table lists those foods which are lowest in calories, from the least up to 100 calories.

*Refer page 59 for average daily protein requirements.

FOOD ENERGY (1)

AVAILABILITY RANGE IN EDIBLE FOODS – FROM THE HIGHEST DOWN

Measured in Calories per 100 gram portion.

Cod Liver Oil	900	Sugar Cane crystals – brown	366
Lard & Dripping	900	Coconut – fresh meat	364
Oils – vegetable, refined	884	Flour – wheat, self-raising	364
Butter – unsalted	727	Flour – wheat, white, fortified	364
Butter – salted	727	Cream from Cows' Milk	364
Margarine – Table	727	Tapioca – dry	363
Margarine – Cooking	720	Chickpeas (Garbanzos)–dry, raw	360
Macadamia Nut kernels – raw	691	Flour – Wheat, white	360
Pecan Nut kernels – raw	687	Rice – Unpolished, raw	359
Coconut – dry meat shredded	672	Sago – dry	358
Bacon – grilled	661	Semolina – dry	358
Brazil Nut kernels – raw	654	Rice – Polished, raw	357
Walnut kernels – raw	648	Corn Meal – dry	355
Pinon (Pinenut) kernels – raw	635	Lamb Chops – medium broiled	355
Hazelnut kernels – raw	634	Soya Grits – "low fat"	355
Safflower Seed kernels – raw	615	Barley – pearled, dry	354
Almond kernels – natural, raw	598	Bulghur Wheat	354
Pistachio Nut kernels – raw	594	Haricot Beans – dry, raw	352
Sesame Seeds – hulled, raw	582	Whey Powder – dry	349
Peanuts – roasted, with skins	580	Maple Sugar – pure	348
Peanuts – raw, without skins	567	Eggs (hen) – yolk, raw	347
Sesame Seeds – whole, raw	563	Cream, Cheese	345
Cashew Nut kernels – raw	561	Flour – Wheat, wholemeal	344
Sunflower Seed kernels – raw	560	Pasta, wholemeal – dry	344
Pignolia (Pinenut) kernels – raw	553	Bananas – dehydrated	340
Pepitas – raw shelled	553	Mung Beans – dry, raw	340
Chocolate – plain milk	538	Wheat, soft – flaked & rolled	340
Chocolate – plain dark	534	Lima Beans – dry, raw	399
Linseed – whole, raw	498	Broadbeans – dry, raw	338
Beef Steak (T-bone)–"well done"	437	Lentils, Brown – dry, raw	336
Pork Chops – broiled "well done"	436	Buckwheat – raw	335
Soya Milk – dry	423	Rye – whole grain	334
Soya Flour – "full fat"	419	Buckwheat flour	333
Soya Beans – dry, raw	403	Wheat, hard red – raw whole	330
Cheese, Cheddar – natural	402	Millet – whole grain	327
Sugar Cane crystals – refined	390	Flour – Rye (100%)	327
Ham – deboned, cooked	389	Wheat, soft std.–raw whole	326
Rolled Oats – dry	388	Honey	322
Sugar Cane Crystals – raw	385	Yeast, Bakers' – dry active	303
Wheat Germ – dry	380	Apples – dried	289
Cheese, Swiss – natural	378	Tuna – canned in oil	288
Gluten Flour	378	Yeast, Brewers'	283
Chestnuts – dried	377		
"Cornflakes" – dry	370	Raisins – dried	279
Pasta, White – dry	367	Yeast, Torula	277

Continued next page

Rice Bran — dry, raw	276	Salmon — baked	182
Dates, Calif. — natural, dry	274	Carob Powder — dry	180
Currants — dried	273	Avocadoes — Fuerte	171
Figs — dried	270	Miso	171
Pears — dried	270	Tuna — canned in water	167
Liver — floured & fried	269	Avocadoes — average	161
Apricots — dried	265	Eggs (hen) — whole, raw	160
Peaches — dried	263	Sweet Potatoes — baked	141
Beef Steak (T-bone) — "rare"	258	Liver — raw	139
Prunes — dried	255	Garlic cloves — raw	137
Chicken — fried	253	Soya Beans — fresh	134
Maple Syrup — pure	252	Lima Beans — boiled	130
Bread — White	243	Soya Beans — boiled	130
Bread — Brown	242	Haricot Beans — boiled	120
Bread — Mixed Grain	240	Rice, Unpolished — boiled	120
Bread — Light Rye	238	Pasta, White — boiled	114
Bread — Dark Rye	237	Sweet Potatoes — raw	114
Bread — Cracked Wheat	235	Sweet Potatoes — boiled	114
Bread — Wholemeal	230	Scallops — steamed	112
Wheat Bran — dry, raw	225	Lentils, Brown — boiled	110
Molasses — "Blackstrap"	213	Rice, Polished — boiled	107
Olives, Green — fresh	211	Breadfruit — raw	106
Veal Chops — medium **broiled**	206	Cheese, Cottage — creamed	106
Flounder — baked	202	Broadbeans — fresh, raw	105
Chicken — roasted	199	Bream fish — steamed	101
Chicken — boiled	198	Cheese, Ricotta	100
Chestnuts — fresh, raw	194		

_87_

FOOD ENERGY (2)

AVAILABILITY RANGE IN EDIBLE FOODS — FROM THE LOWEST UP

Measured in Calories per 100 gram portion

Zucchinis — boiled	12	Lime juice — fresh	28
Vinegar, Malt — distilled	12	Swiss Chard — boiled	28
Cucumbers — peeled, raw	13	Turnips — boiled	28
Cucumbers — whole, raw	14	Turnips — raw	29
Cabbage, Chinese — raw	14	Kohlrabi — raw	29
Vinegar, Apple Cider — filtered	14	Limes — peeled, raw	29
Squash, Summer — boiled	15	Beans (long green) — boiled	30
Celery — boiled	17	Butternut Squash — boiled	30
Lettuce — raw	17	Carrots — boiled	30
Radish — raw	17	Swiss Chard — raw	30
Rhubarb — raw	17	Beets — boiled	31
Zucchinis — raw	17	Cabbage, Red — raw	31
Beet Greens — boiled	18	Beans (long green) — raw	32
Celery — raw	18	Lemons — peeled, raw	32
Squash, Summer — raw	18	Okras — boiled	32
Eggplant — boiled	19	Pumpkins — boiled	33
Asparagus — boiled	20	Honeydew Melons — raw	34
Tomato juice — canned	20	Okras — raw	34
Asparagus — raw	21	Swedes — boiled	34
Watercress — raw	21	Broccoli — raw	35
Cabbage, White — boiled	22	Mung Beans — sprouted	35
Coconut — fresh milk	22	Onions, mature — raw	35
Mushrooms — raw	22	Carrots — raw	36
Tomatoes — ripe, raw	22	Rutabagas — raw	36
Spinach — raw	23	Grapefruit juice — fresh	36
Beet Greens — raw	24	Grapefruit — peeled, raw	37
Cauliflower — boiled	24	Artichokes, Globe — boiled	37
Kohlrabi — boiled	24	Strawberries — raw	37
Canteloupes — raw	25	Brussel Sprouts — boiled	38
Chayotes — boiled	25	Buttermilk	38
Eggplant — raw	25	Soya Milk— reconstituted	38
Spinach — boiled	25	Leeks — boiled	38
Bell Peppers — raw	26	Butternut Pumpkins — raw	39
Broccoli — boiled	26	Artichokes, Globe — raw	40
Cabbage, White — raw	26	Beets —raw	40
Cauliflower — raw	26	Squash, Winter — boiled	40
Lemon juice — fresh	26	Papayas— raw	41
Pumpkins — raw	26	Peaches — raw	41
Tomatoes — boiled	26	Apple juice — canned	42
Whey — liquid	26	Gooseberries — raw	43
Onions, mature — boiled	27	Leeks — raw	43
Watermelons — raw	27	Orange juice — fresh	43
Chives — raw	28	Apricots — raw	45
Chayotes — raw	28	Onions, young — raw	45
		Oranges — peeled, raw	45

Continued next page

Squash, Winter – raw	45	Mangoes – raw	66
Soya Beans – sprouted	46	Pomegranates – raw	66
Tangarines — peeled, raw	46	Milk, Cows' – whole	67
Brussel Sprouts – raw	49	Milk, Goats' – whole	67
Eggs (hen) – white, raw	49	Artichokes, Jerusalem – raw	68
Pineapple juice – canned	49	Oysters – raw	68
Butternut Squash — baked	50	Milk, Human – whole	69
Currants, Red – raw	51	Parsnips – raw	70
Pineapples – raw	52	Peas, fresh – boiled	70
Apples – peeled, raw	53	Shallot bulbs – raw	72
Rolled Oats – boiled	55	Prunes – fresh, raw	75
Parsley – raw	55	Figs – fresh, raw	76
Yogurt from Skimmed Cows' Milk	55	Persimmons – raw	76
Loquats – raw	56	Potatoes – raw or boiled	76
Pears – raw	56	Prune juice – canned	77
Apples – with peel, raw	57	Yogurt, Cows' – whole milk	78
Apricot nectar – canned	57	Peas, fresh – raw	80
Quinces – raw	57	Corn, Sweet – boiled	83
Raspberries, Red – raw	57	Yeast, Bakers' – compressed	86
Blackberries – raw	58	Bananas – ripe, raw	87
Currants, Black – raw	59	Cheese, Cottage – uncreamed	91
Plums – raw	59	Passionfruit – raw	91
Loganberries – raw	60	Peppers, Mature Hot Red – raw	93
Cherries – raw	61	Potatoes – baked	93
Grape juice – canned	62	Yams – boiled	94
Nectarines – raw	62	Custard Apples – raw	96
Guavas – fresh	63	Yams – raw	96
Lychees – raw	64	Corn, Sweet – raw	97
Parsnips – boiled	65	Cheese, Ricotta	100
Grapes – raw	66		

Total Carbohydrates

The most prolific nutrient group in food science is that of the carbohydrates. All chemicals within this group contain varying proportions of carbon, hydrogen and oxygen and include those nutrients we know as starches, sugars and fibers (cellulose).

Carbohydrates are found primarily in foods of plant origin. As starches and sugars, they are readily metabolised by the body, but such assimilation is not the role of fiber. Until comparatively recently, the role of fiber in foodstuffs was virtually ignored. However, research has revealed that such ignorance has, in many cases, led to uncomfortable pathological conditions, especially constipation.

Very few foods of animal origin contain carbohydrates. Small quantities are to be found in eggs and some shellfish. Milk offers larger amounts of carbohydrate in the form of lactose (milk sugar), which accounts for nearly one-third of the solid matter in milk. As a consequence, most cheese contain small quantities of carbohydrate.

The method used to determine total carbohydrate content in foods is known as "carbohydrate by difference". It involves the deduction of water, protein, fat and ash percentages (previously determined) from 100%, representing the edible portion of each food. The resulting figure is universally accepted as the most reliable guide to the carbohydrate content of each food, thereby also affording the best mode of comparison.

Heading the list of foods richest in carbohydrate are the refined (white) crystals of cane (or beet) sugar. As most nutritionists acknowledge, sugar can hardly be regarded as a food, for it is devoid of the nutritional properties necessary to the sustaining of life. However, its inclusion is beneficial for purposes of comparison.

It is true that carbohydrates eaten in excess of the body's needs often induce an accumulation of excess body weight. For this reason, many people seek a diet of foods which are low in carbohydrate. To assist in this regard, total carbohydrates are covered by two graduated lists, the first showing food contents from the highest concentrations of carbohydrate down to 13.0%, the second showing foods graduated from no carbohydrate content up to 13.0%. They are all expressed in grams per 100 grams of edible portion of each food, thus effectively providing the percentage content.

Fiber

Fiber is the cellulose or "roughage" in foodstuffs, a natural component of all unrefined foods of plant origin. It does not enter into the assimilation of the food, but we know that small quantities of dietary fiber are vital to the comfortable and efficient elimination of food residues. Fiber is often referred to as "bulk" in foods, for its role is to provide important roughage to facilitate comfortable and natural bowel movements of food residues.

Refined and processed foods, such as white flour and those products cooked from it, most packaged breakfast "cereals" and many canned food are noticeably deficient in dietary fiber. Animal meats, offal and processed animal foods (such as sausages), refined sugar, sea foods, milk and milk products, vegetable and animal oils, are completely devoid of natural fiber. Consequently, diets comprising 50% or more of these foods can, and usually do, create elimination problems which many people ignore until chronic constipation sets in. The natural remedy is not to take laxatives, for this habit only further weakens the colon without remedying the cause. Dietary correction is the only permanent answer to constipation — include plenty of fresh fruit and vegetables, plus raw nuts and seeds and whole grains.

Fiber content in foods is included in the following list of total carbohydrates, being an important part of the total carbohydrate value of foodstuffs. However, special emphasis has recently been accorded the role of fiber, since it has been realised that many people suffer from constipation due to its lack in their diet. Thus, with the assistance of the United States Department of Agriculture researchers, the following table of fiber in foods has been compiled.

In general, grains, beans, seeds and dried fruits possess highest quantities of fiber, although a few fresh fruits are found surprisingly high on the list, such as guavas, blackberries, red currants and custard apples. As these fruits are also high in moisture, they are consequently the richest sources of food fiber. Rice and wheat brans analyse to contain the highest concentrations of fiber, but they are both extracts of the grain and both very dry, necessitating some moisture to help them become palatable.

As whole foods, buckwheat, followed by dried pears and figs, offer the best nutritional sources of food fiber. If those people seeking added fiber in their diets recognised these facts, more interest would be directed towards whole foods instead of fragmented part-foods, with improvement to the diet in general.

The graduated list on pages 96-7 shows measurements of fiber as grams per 100 grams of a food's edible portion, thereby supplying actual percentage concentrations in each food. Many foods will be seen to be excluded from the list, implying they contain less than 1.3% fiber. Such exclusions embrace all foods of animal origin, together with some fresh fruits and vegetables (which possess some fiber, but less than 1.3%).

TOTAL CARBOHYDRATES (1)

CONTENT RANGE IN EDIBLE FOODS – FROM THE HIGHEST DOWN

Measured in grams per 100 gram portion

Sugar Cane Crystals – refined	99.9	Chocolate – Plain, dark	62.6
Sugar Cane Crystals – raw	99.4	Lima Beans – dry, raw	62.2
Sugar Cane cyrstals – brown	93.8	Wheat Bran – dry, raw	62.1
Sago – dry	90.8	Lentils, Brown – dry, raw	61.7
Maple Sugar – pure	90.0	Chickpeas (Garbanzos) – dry, raw	61.0
Tapioca – dry	88.7	Mung Beans – dry, raw	60.3
Bananas – dehydrated	88.6	Broadbeans – dry, raw	58.2
"Cornflakes" – dry	84.9	Chocolate – Plain, milk	56.4
Rice – Polished, raw	81.0	Molasses – "Blackstrap"	55.0
Carob Powder – dry	80.7	Rice Bran – dry, raw	50.8
Honey	80.0	Bread – white	49.9
Barley – pearled, dry	79.1	Wheat Germ – dry, raw	49.5
Semolina – dry	78.1	Bread – Light Rye	49.1
Chestnuts – dried	78.6	Bread – Dark Rye	48.8
Rice – Unpolished, raw	78.4	Bread – Mixed Grain	48.0
Pasta, White – dry	76.8	Gluten Flour	47.2
		Bread – Wholemeal	46.7
Wheat, soft – flaked & rolled	76.2	Bread – Cracked Wheat	46.7
Bulghur Wheat	75.7	Chestnuts – fresh	42.1
Apples – dried	75.2	Yeast, Bakers' – dry, active	41.5
Flour – Wheat, self-raising	74.9	Soya Milk – dry	40.1
Flour – Wheat, white fortified	74.9	Yeast, Brewers'	38.4
Raisins – dried	74.9	Linseed – whole, raw	37.2
Flour – Wheat, white	73.9	Yeast, Torula	37.0
Corn Meal – dry	73.7	Soya Beans – dry, raw	33.5
Whey Powder – dry	73.5	Sweet Potatoes (yellow) – baked	32.5
Rye – whole grain	73.4	Soya Grits – "low fat"	31.6
Flour – Rye (100%)	73.4	Garlic cloves – raw	30.8
Buckwheat – raw	72.9	Cashew Nut kernels – raw	29.3
Dates, Calif. – natural, dry	72.9	Coconut – dry meat shredded	29.0
Millet – whole grain	72.9	Sweet Potatoes (yellow) – boiled	26.3
Currants – dried	72.8	Sweet Potatoes (yellow) – raw	26.3
Wheat, soft – raw, whole	72.1	Breadfruit – raw	25.2
Buckwheat flour	72.0	Rice – Unpolished, boiled	25.2
Flour – Wheat, wholemeal	71.6	Lima Beans – boiled	24.6
Pasta, Wholemeal – dry	71.6	Rice – Polished, boiled	24.4
Pears – dried	70.0	Soya Flour – "full fat"	24.3
Rolled Oats – dry	69.9	Haricot Beans – boiled	24.0
Figs – dried	69.8	Custard Apples – raw	23.7
Wheat, hard red – whole, raw	69.1	Miso	23.5
Peaches – dried	68.5	Pasta, White – boiled	23.2
Apricots – dried	68.3	Yams – raw	22.6
Prunes – dried	67.4	Bananas – ripe, raw	22.5
Maple Syrup – pure	65.0	Yams – boiled	22.3
Haricot Beans – dry, raw	64.2	Sesame Seeds – whole, raw	21.6

Continued next page

96

TOTAL CARBOHYDRATES (1) continued

Peanuts – roasted, with skins	21.3	Macadamia Nut kernels – raw	15.9
Passionfruit – raw	21.2	Plums – raw	15.6
Potatoes – baked in skin	21.1	Peas, fresh – raw	15.5
Corn, Sweet – raw	21.0	Parsnips – boiled	15.3
Pinon (Pinenut) kernels – raw	20.5	Cherries – raw'	15.1
Lentils, Brown – boiled	20.3	Currants, Black – raw	15.0
Sunflower Seed kernels – raw	19.9	Guavas – fresh	15.0
Prunes – fresh, raw	19.7	Pepitas – raw	15.0
Persimmons – raw	19.3	Quinces – raw	15.0
Pistachio Nut kernels – raw	19.0	Walnut kernels – raw	14.9
Almond kernels – natural, raw	18.9	Apricot nectar – canned	14.6
Figs – fresh, raw	18.9	Pecan Nut kernels – raw	14.6
Peppers, Mature Hot Red – raw	18.1	Pears – raw	14.5
Broadbeans – fresh, raw	17.8	Loganberries – raw	14.4
Sesame Seeds – hulled, raw	17.6	Loquats – raw	14.4
Peanuts – raw, without skins	17.5	Apples – with peel; raw	14.2
Mangoes – raw	17.2	Coconut – fresh meat	14.1
Pomegranates – raw	17.1	Liver – floured and fried	14.0
Potatoes – raw or boiled	17.1	Raspberries, Red – raw	13.9
Grapes – raw or juice	16.8	Apples – peeled, raw	13.8
Shallot bulbs – raw	16.8	Peas, fresh – boiled	13.5
Artichokes, Jerusalem – raw	16.7	Pineapples – raw	13.5
Hazelnut kernels – raw	16.7	Yeast, Bakers' – compressed	13.3
Nectarines – raw	16.5	Pineapple juice – canned	13.2
Lychees – raw	16.4	Soya Beans – fresh	13.2
Parsnips – raw	16.4		

CONTENT RANGE IN EDIBLE FOODS – FROM THE LOWEST UP

Measured in grams per 100 gram portion

Beef Steaks – **broiled**	0
Fish (all) – raw, steamed or baked	0
Cheese, Cheddar – natural	0
Cheese, Swiss – natural	0
Poultry – raw, boiled or roasted	0
Cod Liver Oil	0
Ham – deboned, cooked	0
Lard & Dripping	0
Oils – Vegetable, refined	0
Pork Chops – grilled	0
Scallops – steamed	0
Tuna – canned in water or oil	0
Margarine – Table	.6
Eggs (hen) – yolk, raw	.6
Eggs (hen) – whole, raw	.7
Eggs (hen) – white, raw	.7
Butter – salted or unsalted	.7
Margarine – cooking	.8
Olives, Green – fresh	1.8
Cheese, Cottage – uncreamed	2.4
Cheese, Ricotta	2.5
Zucchinis – boiled	2.5
Cabbage, Chinese – raw	2.6
Bacon – grilled	2.7
Cheese, Cottage – creamed	2.9
Chicken – fried	2.9
Lettuce – raw	3.0
Cream from Cows' Milk	3.0
Celery – boiled	3.1
Cucumbers – peeled, raw	3.1
Watercress – raw	3.2
Beet Greens – boiled	3.3
Cream Cheese	3.4
Cucumbers – whole, raw	3.4
Squash, Summer – boiled	3.5
Asparagus – boiled	3.6
Radishes – raw	3.6
Soya Milk – reconstituted	3.6
Zucchinis – raw	3.6
Spinach – boiled	3.7
Asparagus – raw	3.8
Mushrooms – raw	3.8
Celery – raw	3.9

Rhubarb – raw	3.9
Squash, Summer – raw	4.0
Spinach – raw	4.1
Eggplant – boiled	4.1
Tomato juice – canned	4.1
Oysters – raw	4.1
Buttermilk	4.2
Cauliflower – boiled	4.2
Cabbage, White – boiled	4.3
Cauliflower – raw	4.6
Beet Greens – raw	4.6
Cows' Milk – whole	4.6
Goats' Milk – whole	4.6
Coconut – fresh milk	4.7
Tomatoes – ripe, raw	4.7
Swiss Chard – boiled	4.8
Broccoli – boiled	4.9
Liver – raw	5.0
Vinegar, Distilled – malt	5.0
Whey – liquid	5.1
Kohlrabi – boiled	5.3
Swiss Chard – raw	5.3
Soya Beans – sprouted	5.3
Cabbage, White – raw	5.4
Eggplant – raw	5.5
Tomatoes – boiled	5.5
Bell Peppers –raw	5.6
Canteloupes – raw	5.7
Yogurt from whole Cows' Milk	5.7
Chives – raw	5.8
Vinegar, Apple Cider – filtered	5.9
Avocadoes – Fuerte	6.0
Kohlrabi – raw	6.1
Onions, mature – boiled	6.1
Turnips – boiled	6.2
Avocadoes – average	6.3
Broccoli – raw	6.3
Beans (long green) – boiled	6.4
Chayotes – boiled	6.4
Turnips – raw	6.4
Pumpkins – raw	6.5
Watermelons – raw	6.5
Brussel Sprouts – boiled	6.6
Mung Beans – sprouted	6.6
Beans (long green) – raw	6.8

Continued next page

Butternut Squash – boiled	6.9	Artichokes, Globe – boiled	9.9
Cabbage, Red – raw	6.9	Parsley – raw	10.0
Pumpkins – boiled	6.9	Oats, rolled – boiled	10.0
Yogurt from skimmed Cows' Milk	6.9	Squash, Winter – raw	10.4
Beets – boiled	7.0	TVP – hydrated	10.4
Carrots – boiled	7.0	Onions, young – raw	10.5
Chayotes – raw	7.0	Papayas — raw	10.5
Okras – boiled	7.2	Artichokes, Globe – raw	10.6
Human Milk – whole	7.4	Orange juice – fresh	10.6
Okras – raw	7.5	Gooseberries – raw	10.7
Leeks – boiled	8.0	Peaches – raw	10.7
Lemon juice – fresh	8.0	Corn, Sweet – boiled	10.8
Rutabagas – boiled	8.0	Soya Beans – boiled	10.8
Honeydew Melons – raw	8.1	Brazil Nut kernels – raw	10.9
Onions, mature – raw	8.2	Oranges – peeled, raw	11.1
Grapefruit juice – fresh	8.5	**Tangarines** – peeled, raw	11.2
Carrots – raw	8.6	Apricots – raw	11.4
Strawberries – raw	8.6	Apple juice – canned	11.5
Rutabagas– raw	8.6	Pignolia (pinenut) kernels – raw	11.6
Brussel Sprouts – raw	8.7	Butternut **Squash** – baked	11.7
Squash, Winter – boiled	9.0	Limes – peeled, raw	11.9
Leeks – raw	9.1	Safflower Seed kernels – raw	12.4
Grapefruit – peeled, raw	9.2	Currants, Red	12.5
Beets– raw	9.3	Blackberries – raw	12.7
Butternut **Squash– raw**	9.4		

FIBRE

CONTENT RANGE IN EDIBLE FOODS – FROM THE HIGHEST DOWN

Measured in grams per 100 gram portion

Rice Bran – dry, raw	11.5	Soya Flour – "full fat"	2.3
Wheat Bran – dry, raw	10.3	Wheat – all varieties, whole	2.3
Buckwheat – raw	9.9	Broadbeans – fresh, raw	2.2
Peppers, Mature Hot Red – raw	9.0	Wheat, soft – flaked & rolled	2.2
Linseed – whole, raw	8.8	Peas, fresh – raw or boiled	2.1
Carob Powder – dry	7.7	Bananas – dehydrated	2.0
Broadbeans – dry, raw	6.7	Parsnips – raw or boiled	2.0
Pears – dried	6.4	Rye – whole grain	2.0
Sesame Seeds – whole, raw	6.3	Soya Milk – dry	2.0
Figs – dried	5.6	Gooseberries – raw	1.9
Guavas – fresh	5.6	Peanuts – raw, without skins	1.9
Chickpeas (Garbanzos)–dry, raw	5.0	Pistachio Nut kernels – raw	1.9
Soya Beans – dry, raw	4.9	Pepitas – raw shelled	1.9
Soya Grits – "low fat"	4.6	Butternut Squash – baked	1.8
Mung Beans – dry, raw	4.4	Parsley – raw	1.8
Lima Beans – dry, raw	4.3	Bulghur Wheat	1.7
Blackberries – raw	4.1	Lima Beans – boiled	1.7
Coconut – fresh meat	4.1	Quinces – raw	1.7
Coconut – dry meat shredded	4.0	Walnut kernels – raw	1.7
Lentils, Brown – dry, raw	4.0	Yeast, Brewers'	1.7
Sunflower Seed kernels	3.8	Avocados – Average	1.6
Currants, Red – raw	3.5	Brussel Sprouts – raw or boiled	1.6
Yeast, Torula	3.3	Buckwheat flour	1.6
Custard Apples – raw	3.2	Corn Meal – dry	1.6
Millet – whole grain	3.2	Persimmons – raw	1.6
Apples – dried	3.1	Prunes – dried	1.6
Brazil Nut kernels – raw	3.1	Soya Beans – boiled	1.6
Peaches – dried	3.1	Avocadoes – Fuerte	1.5
Raspberries, Red – raw	3.1	Broccoli – raw or boiled	1.5
Apricots – dried	3.0	Capsicums – raw	1.5
Hazelnut kernels – raw	3.0	Garlic cloves – raw	1.5
Loganberries – raw	3.0	Squash, Winter – raw or boiled	1.4
Wheat Germ – dry, raw	2.9	Butternut Squash – raw or boiled	1.4
Currants, Black – raw	2.8	Cashew Nut kernels – raw	1.4
Peanuts – roasted, with skins	2.8	Soya Beans – fresh	1.4
Almond kernels – natural, raw	2.6	Beet Greens – raw	1.3
Chestnuts – dried	2.5		
Macadamia Nut kernels – raw	2.5		
Artichokes, Globe – raw or boiled	2.4	
Sesame Seeds – hulled, raw	2.4	
Dates, Calif. – natural, dry	2.3	
Flour – Wheat, wholemeal	2.3	
Miso	2.3	
Pasta – Wholemeal, dry	2.3	
Pecan Nut kernels – raw	2.3	

AVERAGE FIBRE CONTENT NOT AVAILABLE (NA) –
but these goods are known to contain more than one gram per 100 gram portion:

Haricot Beans – raw or boiled
Safflower Seed kernels
Yeast, Bakers' – dry or compressed

Minerals

Minerals from edible foods are essential to the human body. They help to form its essential structure and vitally assist the body's normal functioning. Chemically, minerals are of comparatively simple structure and are employed in the body in varying, small amounts.

Minerals required by the body are chemical compounds composed of various elements. Determination of the mineral content of foods is actually made by analysis of the mineral elements. It is these elements which are listed in all food analysis tables and this book is no exception.

The body's requirements of different elements varies over a very considerable range. In order, oxygen is the most needed element, followed by carbon, hydrogen and nitrogen. Then we come to the elements which are specifically indicative of the mineral content of foods.

In order of graduated quantities are calcium, phosphorus, potassium, sulphur, chlorine, flourine, magnesium, iron, manganese, silicon, copper, sodium, iodine, zinc and cobalt. By this time, we are well into the trace elements and, although many more in diminishing quantities are on record, insufficient research on them has been completed to permit their inclusion in this book. Indeed, it is to be hoped that a further edition of this book will be able to include at least zinc, copper and iodine. Our prime concern is now to offer tables of quantities of major researched nutrients in graduated lists as guides to dietary selection.

To this extent, the six mineral elements represented are calcium, phosphorus, iron, sodium, potassium and magnesium. All are alkaline-forming (in terms of their digestive ash residues), with the exception of phosphorus, itself being acid-forming.

The figures given for calcium and magnesium might not accurately represent the amount of actual availability in a particular food. They will always represent the measured content of these elements in the food, but some might be chemically bound to oxalic acid. If so, highly insoluble compounds are formed which the body cannot appropriate. They are excreted as insoluble oxalites or, if in large quantities, are retained in the kidneys where they form "stones" or "gravel". Foods with excessive amounts of oxalic acid should be eaten with care as they deprive the body of some of its store of these two vital elements. Such depleting foods are animal meats, chocolate, coffee, tea, beet greens, spinach, rhubarb and silverbeet. Also containing oxalic acid, but with an abundance of calcium and magnesium to handle it, are peanuts, wheat germ, almonds, cashew nuts, parsley, beets, limes, celery, raspberries, okra and sweet potatoes.

Most mineral elements suffer losses during cooking, especially when boiled. Potassium is especially highly soluble and suffers most losses from cooking. Sodium is next most affected. It will be noticed that the tables for sodium are divided into two groups — those foods which have added sodium, in the form of common salt (sodium chloride), are separated from the foods possessing natural sodium, thereby giving a more accurate guide to the occurence of this mineral in its two major forms and to guide those people who have recognized the dangers of consuming too much common salt in ther diet.

All tables of mineral contents in foods show values in milligrams per 100 gram edible portion of the food and all are graduated from the highest. Each table contains foods in descending order of richness of each mineral element for which a sufficient number of foods have been analysed.

CALCIUM

CONTENT RANGE IN EDIBLE FOODS – FROM THE HIGHEST DOWN

Measured in milligrams per 100 gram portion

Sesame Seeds – whole, raw	1160	Sugar Cane crystals – brown	100
Cheese, Swiss – natural	950	Beet Greens – boiled	99
Cheese, Cheddar – natural	860	Broccoli – boiled	98
Molasses – "Blackstrap"	684	Cheese, Cottage – creamed	94
Whey Powder – dry	646	Cheese, Cottage – uncreamed	93
Yeast, Torula	424	Flour – Wheat, self-raising	93
Carob powder – dry	352	Spinach – boiled	92
Soya Milk – dry	330	Currants – dried	90
Chocolate – Plain milk	295	Oysters – raw	88
Linseed – whole, raw	271	Okras – raw	87
Parsley – raw	260	Apricots – dried	84
Soya Grits – "low fat"	252	Walnut kernels – raw	84
Almond kernels – natural, raw	245	Cream from Cows' Milk	82
Figs – dried	240	Wheat Germ – dry, raw	81
Soya Beans – dry, raw	226	Okras – boiled	80
Yeast, Brewers'	210	Rice Bran – dry, raw	76
Hazelnut kernels – raw	209	Bread – Light Rye	75
Soya Flour – "full fat"	205	Peanuts – roasted with skins	73
Watercress – raw	192	Pecan Nut kernels – raw	73
Brazil Nut kernels – raw	186	Soya Beans – boiled	73
Chickpeas (Garbanzos) – dry, raw	150	Chives – raw	69
Yogurt from whole Cows' Milk	147	Flounder – baked	69
Haricot Beans – dry, raw	146	Lima Beans – dry, raw	69
Maple Sugar – pure	143	Miso	68
Yogurt from skimmed Cows' Milk	140	Raisins – dried	68
Onions, young – raw	136	Soya Beans – fresh	67
Eggs (hen) – yolk, raw	131	Bread – Dark Rye	62
Pistachio Nut kernels – raw	131	Dates, Calif. – natural, dry	59
Goats' Milk – whole	129	Lentils, Brown – dry, raw	58
Broccoli – raw	123	Rutabagas – raw	58
Sunflower Seed kernels – raw	120	Peanuts – raw, without skins	57
Beet Greens – raw	119	Leeks – raw	56
Mung Beans – dry, raw	118	Rolled Oats – dry	55
Buttermilk	115	Rutabagas – boiled	55
Cows' Milk – whole	115	Eggs (hen) – whole, raw	54
Scallops – steamed	115	Leeks – boiled	54
Swiss Chard – raw	115	Parsnips – raw	54
Buckwheat – raw	114		53
Sesame Seeds – hulled, raw	110	Chestnuts – dried	52
Swiss Chard – boiled	105	Artichokes, Globe – raw or boiled	51
Wheat Bran – dry, raw	105	Prunes – dried	51
Maple Syrup – pure	104	Pepitas – raw, shelled	51
Broadbeans – dry, raw	102	Whey – liquid	51
Rhubarb – raw	101	Haricot Beans – boiled	50
Spinach – raw	101	Kohlrabi – raw	50

Continued next page

CALCIUM continued

Parsnips — boiled	50	Sweet Potatoes — raw or boiled	32
Currants, Black — raw	49	Lemons — peeled, raw	31
Figs — fresh, raw	49	Milk, Human — whole	31
Turnips — raw	49	Onions, mature — raw	31
Beans (long green) — raw	48	Brussel Sprouts — boiled	30
Celery — raw	48	Radishes — raw	30
Macadamia Nut kernels — raw	48	Soya Milk — recon.	30
Soya Beans — sprouted	48		
Cabbage, White — raw	47		
Turnips — boiled	47		
Beans (long green) — boiled	46		
Cabbage, Chinese — raw	46		
Cabbage, White — boiled	43		
Cabbage, Red — raw	42		
Wheat, soft — whole, raw	42		
Yeast, Bakers' — dry, active	42		
Blackberries — raw	41		
Kohlrabi — boiled	41		
Carrots — raw	40		
Cream Cheese	40		
Gluten Flour	40		
Limes — peeled, raw	40		
Peaches — dried	40		
Sweet Potatoes — baked	40		
Oranges — peeled, raw	39		
Cashew Nut kernels — raw	38		
Celery — boiled	38		
Rye — whole grain	38		
Chocolate — Plain dark	37		
Flour — Wheat, wholemeal	37		
Mandarins — peeled, raw	37		
Pasta, Wholemeal — dry	37		
Shallot bulbs — raw	37		
Carrots — boiled	36		
Raspberries, Red — raw	36		
Wheat, hard red — whole, raw	36		
Wheat, soft — flaked & rolled	36		
Bread — Cracked Wheat	35		
Bread — Wholemeal	35		
Bream fish — steamed	35		
Loganberries — raw	35		
Pears — dried	34		
Breadfruit — raw	33		
Buckwheat flour	33		
Currants, Red — raw	33		
Bananas — dehydrated	32		
Brussel Sprouts — raw	32		
Lettuce — raw	32		
Orange juice — fresh	32		

AVERAGE CALCIUM CONTENT NOT AVAILABLE (NA) —
but these foods are known to contain more than 30 milligrams per 100 gram portion:

Bread — Mixed Grain
Cheese, Ricotta
Safflower Seed kernels — raw
TVP — hydrated

PHOSPHORUS

CONTENT RANGE IN EDIBLE FOODS — FROM THE HIGHEST DOWN

Measured in milligrams per 100 gram portion

* Yeast, Brewers'	1753	* Lentils, Brown — dry, raw	334
Yeast, Torula	1713	* Chickpeas (Garbanzos) — dry, raw	331
Rice Bran — dry, raw	1386	* Beef Steak (T-bone)—"well done"	322
* Yeast, Bakers' — dry, active	1291	Millet — whole grain	311
Wheat Bran — dry, raw	1223	Haricot Beans — dry, raw	309
Pepitas — raw, shelled	1144	Miso	309
Wheat Germ — dry, raw	990	Tuna — canned in oil	294
Sunflower Seed kernels — raw	837	Bacon — grilled	292
Brazil Nut kernels — raw	693	* Tuna — canned in water	290
Soya Milk — dry	680	* Pecan Nut kernels — raw	289
Soya Grits — "low fat"	634	Chocolate — Plain dark	287
Sesame Seeds — whole, raw	616	Buckwheat — raw	282
Cheese, Swiss — natural	605	Rice — Unpolished, raw	282
Pinon (Pinenut) kernels — raw	604	* Pork Chops — broiled	275
Soya Flour — "full fat"	593	* Flour — Rye (100%)	269
Sesame Seeds — hulled, raw	592	Chicken — roasted	268
Whey Powder — dry	589	Veal Chops — broiled	267
Soya Beans — dry, raw	554	* Chicken — boiled	265
Eggs (hen) — yolk, raw	553	Corn Meal — dry	256
* Liver — floured & fried	552	* Buckwheat flour	247
Cheese, Cheddar — natural	506	Chicken — fried	247
* Pistachio Nut kernels — raw	500	* Flounder — baked	244
Flour — Wheat, self-raising	484	Chocolate — Plain milk	242
* Almond kernels — natural, raw	473	Bream fish — steamed	238
Linseed — whole, raw	462	* Barley — peeled, dry	228
Walnut kernels — raw	453	Soya Beans — fresh	225
* Salmon — baked	414	* Eggs (hen) — whole, raw	218
* Peanuts — roasted, with skins	404	* Beef Steak (T-bone) — "rare"	209
Peanuts — raw, without skins	400	Garlic Cloves — raw	202
Wheat, soft — whole, raw	400	* Ham — deboned, cooked	192
Yeast, Bakers' — compressed	394	* Cheese, Cottage — uncreamed	182
Broadbeans — dry, raw	391	Coconut — dry meat shredded	180
Lima Beans — dry, raw	385	Soya Beans — boiled	179
Wheat, hard red — whole, raw	383	* Lamb Chops — grilled	165
* Rye — whole grain	376	Chestnuts — dried	162
* Cashew Nut kernels — raw	373	Macadamia Nut kernels — raw	161
Flour — Wheat, wholemeal	372	Pasta, white — dry	161
Pasta, Wholemeal — dry	372	Broadbeans — fresh, raw	157
* Rolled Oats — dry	371	Lima Beans — boiled	154
Wheat, soft — flaked & rolled	342	Cheese, Cottage — creamed	152
Mung Beans — dry, raw	340	Oysters — raw	149
Bulghur Wheat	338	Bread — Light Rye	147
* Scallops — steamed	338	Cream Cheese	140
* Hazelnut kernels — raw	337	Gluten Flour	140
Liver — raw	336		

Continued next page

PHOSPHORUS continued

Currants — dried	138
Peaches — dried	138
Raisins — dried	130
Bread — Dark Rye	124
Haricot Beans — boiled	122
Mushrooms — raw	116
Peas, fresh — raw	116
Corn, Sweet — raw	115
Apricots — dried	114
Rice — Polished, raw	111
Goats' Milk — whole	106
Bananas — dehydrated	102
Figs — dried	101
Lentils, Brown — boiled	101
Peas, fresh — boiled	100
Semolina — dry	100
Yogurt from Cows' Milk	100
Buttermilk	96
Milk, Cows' — whole	96
Coconut — fresh meat	95
Rice, Unpolished — boiled	90
Corn, Sweet — boiled	89
Artichokes, Globe — raw	88
Chestnuts — fresh, raw	88
Flour — Wheat, white fortified	87
Flour — Wheat, white plain	87
Molasses — "Blackstrap"	84
Carob Powder — dry	81
Brussel Sprouts — raw	79
Parsnips — raw	79
Prunes — dried	79
Artichokes, Jerusalem — raw	78
Peppers, Mature Hot Red — raw	78
Broccoli — raw	77
Bread — White Wheat	74
Parsnips — boiled	74
Parsley — raw	72
Brussel Sprouts — boiled	71
Artichokes, Globe — boiled	69
Soya Beans — sprouted	67
Potatoes — baked in skin	65
Cauliflower — raw	64
Mung Beans — sprouted	64
Dates, Calif. — natural, dry	63
Asparagus — raw	62
Soya Milk — recon.	62
Broccoli — boiled	61
Cream from Cows' milk	60
Shallot bulbs — raw	60
Yams — raw	60

AVERAGE PHOSPHORUS CONTENT NOT AVAILABLE (NA) — but these foods are known to contain more than 60 milligrams per 100 gram portion.

Bread — Mixed Grain
Bread — Cracked Wheat
Bread — Brown
Bread — Wholemeal
Cheese, Ricotta
Pignolia (Pinenut) kernels — raw
Safflower Seed kernels — raw
TVP — hydrated

IRON

CONTENT RANGE IN EDIBLE FOODS – FROM THE HIGHEST DOWN

Measured in milligrams per 100 gram portion

Yeast, Bakers' – dry, active	20.5	Brazil Nut kernels – raw	3.4
Rice Bran – dry, raw	19.4	Hazelnut kernels – raw	3.4
Yeast, Torula	19.3	Beet Greens – raw	3.3
Yeast, Brewers'	17.3	Beef Steak (T-bone) – "rare"	3.3
Molasses – "Blackstrap"	16.1	Chestnuts – dried	3.3
Liver– floured & fried	14.2	Spinach – raw	3.3
Wheat Bran – dry, raw	13.5	Flour – wheat, wholemeal	3.2
Pepitas – raw, shelled	11.2	Pasta, Wholemeal – dry	3.2
Sesame Seeds – whole, raw	10.5	Wheat, soft – flaked & rolled	3.2
Liver– raw	10.4	Buckwheat – raw	3.1
Wheat Germ – dry, raw	9.9	Wheat, hard red – whole, raw	3.1
Soya Grits – "low Fat"	9.3	Bread – Wholemeal	3.0
Soya Milk – dry	9.0	Bread – Cracked Wheat	3.0
"Cornflakes" – dry	8.8	Dates, Calif. – natural, dry	3.0
Soya Beans – dry, raw	8.4	Lima Beans – boiled	3.0
Mung Beans – dry, raw	7.7	Scallops – steamed	3.0
Lima Beans – dry, raw	7.6	Spinach– boiled	3.0
Soya Flour – "full fat"	7.4	Flour – White, fortified	2.9
Pistachio Nut kernels – raw	7.3	Pork Chops – broiled	2.9
Lentils, Brown – dry, raw	7.2	Bananas – dehydrated	2.8
Broadbeans – dry, raw	7.1	Buckwheat Flour	2.8
Sunflower Seed kernels –raw	7.1	Olives, Green – fresh	2.8
Chickpeas (Garbanzos) – dry, raw	6.9	Swiss Chard– raw	2.8
Haricot Beans – dry, raw	6.8	Soya Beans – fresh	2.8
Millet – whole grain	6.8	Bacon – grilled	2.7
Parsley – raw	6.5	Peanuts – roasted, with skins	2.7
Eggs (hen) – Yolk, raw	6.2	Flour – Rye (100%)	2.7
Peaches – dried	6.0	Soya Beans – boiled	2.7
Oysters – raw	5.7	Haricot Beans – boiled	2.5
Pinon (Pinenut) kernels – raw	5.2	Swiss Chard– boiled	2.5
Beef Steak (T-bone)–"well done"	5.0	Corn Meal – dry	2.4
Linseed – whole, raw	4.4	Eggs (hen) – whole, raw	2.4
Almond kernels – natural, raw	4.3	Ham – deboned, cooked	2.4
Apricots – dried	4.3	Peanuts – raw, without skin	2.4
Rolled Oats – dry	4.1	Pecan Nut kernels – raw	2.4
Prune juice	4.1	Sesame Seeds – hulled, raw	2.4
Yeast, Bakers' – compressed	4.0	Walnut kernels – raw	2.4
Prunes – dried	3.9	Breadbeans – fresh, raw	2.2
Cashew Nut kernels – raw	3.8	Currants – dried	2.2
Bulghur Wheat	3.7	Lentils, Brown – boiled	2.2
Rye – whole grain	3.7	Raisins – dried	2.2
Veal Chops – medium broiled	3.7	Chicken – fried or roasted	2.1
Coconut – dry meat shredded	3.5	Coconut – fresh meat	2.0
Figs – dried	3.5	Lamb Chops – medium broiled	2.0
Wheat, soft – whole, raw	3.5	Macadamia Nut kernels – raw	2.0

Continued next page

IRON continued

Beet Greens – boiled	1.9	Soya Beans– sprouted	1.0
Chicken – boiled	1.9	Sugar Cane crystals– brown	1.0
Peas, fresh – raw	1.9		
Chocolate – Plain, milk	1.8		
Peas, fresh – boiled	1.8		
Watercress – raw	1.8		
Apples – dried	1.7		
Bread – Brown	1.7		
Chestnuts – fresh	1.7		
Chives – raw	1.7		
Miso	1.7		
Rice – Unpolished, raw	1.7		
Bread – Rye, Dark or Light	1.6		
Tuna – canned in water	1.6		
Garlic Cloves – raw	1.5		
Flounder – baked	1.4		
Flour – Wheat, white	1.4		
Flour – Wheat, self-raising	1.4		
Maple Sugar – pure	1.4		
Artichokes, Globe– raw	1.3		
Broccoli– raw	1.3		
Brussel Sprouts– raw	1.3		
Loganberries– raw	1.3		
Mung Beans– sprouted	1.3		
Passionfruit– raw	1.3		
Pasta, White– dry	1.3		
Breadfruit– raw	1.2		
Currants, Black– raw	1.2		
Maple Syrup– pure	1.2		
Peppers, Mature Hot Red – raw	1.2		
Salmon– boiled	1.2		
Shallot bulbs– raw	1.2		
Tuna– canned in oil	1.2		
Artichokes, Globe– boiled	1.1		
Barley– pearled, dry	1.1		
Cucumbers– whole, raw	1.1		
Leeks– raw	1.1		
Pears– dried	1.1		
Raspberries, Red– raw	1.1		
Asparagus– raw	1.0		
Bread– White Wheat	1.0		
Broccoli– boiled	1.0		
Brussel Sprouts– boiled	1.0		
Currants, Red– raw	1.0		
Leeks– boiled	1.0		
Mushrooms– raw	1.0		
Radishes– raw	1.0		
Semolina– dry	1.0		

AVERAGE IRON CONTENT NOT AVAILABLE (NA) –
but these foods are known to contain more than 1.0 milligrams per 100 gram portion.

Bread – Mixed Grain
Carob Powder – dry
Pignolia (Pinenut) kernels – raw
Safflower Seed kernels– raw
TVP– hydrated

SODIUM

CONTENT RANGE IN EDIBLE FOODS – FROM THE HIGHEST DOWN

Measured in milligrams per 100 gram portion

a) FOODS WITH ADDED SODIUM CHLORIDE (NaCl – Common Salt):

Bacon – grilled	3,328
Miso	2,950
Margarine—Cooking or Table	1,250
Ham – deboned, cooked	1,106
"Cornflakes" – dry	990
Tuna – canned in water	875
Butter – salted	843
Tuna – canned in oil	800
Flour – Wheat, self-raising	730
Cheese, Cheddar – natural	610
Bread – Dark Rye	593
Bread – Light Rye	557
Bread – Brown	538
Bread – Cracked Wheat	529
Bread – Wholemeal	529
Bread – White	507
Soya Milk – dry	500
Cream Cheese	337
Cheese, Cottage – Uncreamed	290
Scallops – steamed	265
Flounder – baked	237
Cheese, Cottage – Creamed	229
Cheese, Swiss – Natural	157
Salmon – baked	116
Bream fish – steamed	113
Oysters – raw	73
Soya Milk—reconstituted	43

b) FOODS WITHOUT ADDED SODIUM CHLORIDE

Eggs (hen) – yolk, raw	564
Veal Chops – medium broiled	214
Eggs (hen) – white, raw	158
Celery – raw	135
Beet Greens– raw	130
Beef Steak (T-bone)–"well done"	126
Chocolate – Plain, milk	125
Eggs (hen) – Whole, raw	122
Yeast, Brewers'	121
Liver– floured & fried	120
Pork Chops – broiled	115

Celery – boiled	98
Chicken – boiled	98
Molasses – "Blackstrap"	96
Chicken – fried	94
Lamb Chops – medium broiled	91
Liver– raw	87
Beef Steak (T-bone) – "rare"	82
Chicken – roasted	79
Beets – raw	78
Spinach– raw	78
Beet Greens – boiled	76
Swiss Chard — raw	72
Spinach– boiled	71
Carrots – raw	65
Cream from Cows' Milk	65
Swiss Chard – boiled	65
Figs – dried	60
Sesame Seeds – whole, raw	60
Buttermilk	56
Cows' Milk – whole	56
Watercress – raw	56

Beets – boiled	52
Yeast, Bakers' – dry, active	52
Raisins – dried	49
Turnips – raw	48
Turnips – boiled	47
Carrots – boiled	46
Artichokes, Globe – raw	43
Haricot Beans – dry, raw	43
Yogurt from Cows' Milk	40
Parsley – raw	39
Sugar Cane Crystals – brown	38
Goats' Milk	34
Lentils, Brown – dry, raw	33
Artichokes, Globe – boiled	30
Sunflower Seed kernels– raw	30
Passionfruit – raw	28
Cabbage, Red – raw	26
Chickpeas (Garbanzos)–dry, raw	26
Coconut – fresh milk	25
Apricots – dried	23
Cabbage, Chinese – raw	23
Cabbage, White – raw	21
Currants – dried	21

Continued next page

Coconut — fresh meat	19	Sweet Potatoes — baked	12
Garlic Cloves — raw	19	Cauliflower — raw	11
Radishes— raw	18	Parsnips — boiled	11
Breadfruit — raw	15	Peaches — dried	11
Broccoli — raw	15	Wheat Bran — dry, raw	11
Cashew Nut kernels — raw	15	Broadbeans— dry, raw	10
Haricot Beans — boiled	15	Broccoli— boiled	10
Yeast, Torula	15	Brussel Sprouts— boiled	10
Cabbage, White — boiled	14	Honey	10
Cherimoyas — raw	14	Maple Syrup— pure	10
Maple Sugar— pure	14	Sweet Potatoes— raw or boiled	10
Human Milk— whole	14	Cauliflower— boiled	9
Brussel Sprouts — raw	13	Cucumbers— whole or peeled	9
Canteloupes— raw	13	Kohlrabi— raw	9
Chocolate — Plain, dark	13	Rice, Unpolished — dry, raw	9
Coconut — dry meat shredded	13	Butter— unsalted	8
Chestnuts — dried	12	Bell Peppers-raw	8
Honeydew Melons— raw	12	Mushrooms— raw	8
Lettuce — raw	12	Onions, Mature— raw	8
Parsnips— raw	12	Prunes— dried	8
Shallot, bulbs — raw	12	Rhubarb— raw	8
Semolina — dry	12	Sugar Cane Crystals— raw	8

AVERAGE SODIUM CONTENT NOT AVAILABLE (NA) — but these foods are known to contain more than 8 milligrams per 100 gram portion.

Bread — Mixed Grain
Carob Powder — dry
Cheese — Ricotta
Chives — raw
Chocolate — Plain dark
Gluten Flour
Lentils, Brown — boiled
Linseed— whole, raw
Macadamia Nut kernels — raw
Pepitas — raw
Peppers, Mature Hot Red — raw
Pistachio Nut kernels — raw
Safflower Seed kernels — raw
Sesame Seeds — hulled raw
TVP — hydrated (has high added NaCl)
Whey— liquid
Whey Powder — dry
Yams — raw or boiled

POTASSIUM

CONTENT RANGE IN EDIBLE FOODS – FROM THE HIGHEST DOWN

Measured in milligrams per 100 gram portion

Molasses – "Blackstrap"	2,927	Beef Steak (T-bone)–"well done"	580
Yeast, Torula	2,046	Custard Apples – raw	578
Yeast, Bakers' – dry, active	1,998	Pears – dried	573
Soya Grits – "low fat"	1,942	Beet Greens – raw	570
Yeast, Brewers'	1,894	Apples – dried	569
Soya Flour – "full fat"	1,730	Parsnips– raw	541
Soya Beans – dry, raw	1,677	Soya Beans – boiled	540
Soya Milk – dry	1,640	Garlic Cloves – raw	529
Apricots – dried	1,561	Swiss Chard — raw	526
Lima Beans – dry, raw	1,499	Parsnips– boiled	505
Rice Bran – dry, raw	1,495	Potatoes – baked in skin	503
Bananas – dehydrated	1,477	Scallops – steamed	496
Haricot Beans – dry, raw	1,194	Walnuts kernels – raw	491
Peaches – dried	1,191	Yeast, Bakers' – compressed	482
Wheat Bran – dry, raw	1,050	Coconut – fresh meat	480
Mung Beans – dry, raw	1,028	Mushrooms – raw	480
Wheat Germ – dry, raw	1,020	Swiss Chard – boiled	480
Pistachio Nut kernels – raw	972	Broadbeans – fresh, raw	471
Sunflower Seed kernels–raw	920	Rye – whole grain	467
Parsley – raw	903	Cashew Nut kernels – raw	464
Figs – dried	900	Bacon – grilled	462
Chestnuts – dried	875	Pork Chops – broiled	458
		Avocadoes – Average	455
Raisins – dried	840	Chestnuts – fresh	454
Olives, Green – fresh	809	Liver– floured & fried	453
Chickpeas (Garbanzos) – dry, raw	797	Buckwheat – raw	448
Almond kernels – natural, raw	773	Salmon – baked	443
Lentils, Brown – dry, raw	757	Breadfruit – raw	439
Sesame Seeds – whole, raw	725	Artichokes, Globe – raw	430
Peanuts – roasted, with skins	720	Millet – whole grain	430
Currants – dried	719	Artichokes, Jerusalem – raw	420
Brazil Nut kernels – raw	715	Brussel Sprouts – raw	420
Hazelnut kernels – raw	704	Coconut – dry meat shredded	420
Peanuts – raw, without skins	700	Chocolate– Plain, milk	413
Spinach– raw	700	Lamb Chops – broiled	410
Prunes – dried	694	Potatoes – raw or boiled	407
Cream Cheese	686	Broccoli – raw	388
Dates, Calif. – natural, dry	648	Kohlrabi – raw	382
Spinach– boiled	637	Wheat, soft – whole, raw	380
Avocadoes – Fuerte	604	Bananas – ripe, raw	377
Pecan Nut kernels – raw	603	Beef Steak (T-bone) – "rare"	377
Lima Beans – boiled	602	Wheat, soft – whole, raw	376
Yams – raw	600	Wheat, hard red – whole, raw	370
Yams – boiled	590	Flour – Wheat, wholemeal	370
Flounder – baked	587	Pasta, Wholemeal – dry	370

Continued next page

POTASSIUM continued

Squash, Winter— raw	369
Chicken — roasted	368
Currants, Black — raw	360
Squash, Winter — boiled	360
Rolled Oats — dry	354
Sugar Cane Crystals — brown	350
Loquats — raw	348
Passionfruit — raw	348
Pumpkins— raw	340
Peas, fresh — raw	338
Miso	334
Shallot bulbs — raw	334
Beet Greens — boiled	332
Celery — raw	332
Leeks — raw	330
Radishes— raw	322
Beets — raw	320
Haricot Beans — boiled	320
Leeks — boiled	320
Tuna — canned in oil	320
Nectarines — raw	307
Carrots— raw	305
Artichokes, Globe— boiled	301
Brussel Sprouts— boiled	300
Watercress— raw	298
Apricots— raw	294
Guavas— fresh	289
Liver — raw	288
Tomatoes— raw	287
Chicken— fried	285
Corn Meal— dry	284
Chocolate— Plain dark	282
Rhubarb— raw	282
Bream fish— steamed	281
Kohlrabi— boiled	278
Tuna— canned in water	275
Beans (long green) — raw	272
Butternut Squash — baked	271
Cabbage, Red— raw	268
Broccoli— boiled	267
Macadamia Nut kernels— raw	264
Canteloupes	263
Corn, Sweet— raw	260
Pomegranates— raw	259
Beans (long green) — boiled	258
Cabbage, Chinese— raw	253
Cabbage, White— raw	250
Chives— raw	250
Turnips— raw	245

Tomatoes— boiled	244
Sweet Potatoes— raw or boiled	243
Maple Sugar— pure	242
Persimmons— raw	242
Lentils, Brown— boiled	240
Pumpkins— boiled	240
Turnips— boiled	240
Celery— boiled	238
Honeydew Melons— raw	235
Okras— raw	235
Prune juice— canned	235
Currants, Red— raw	234
Papayas — raw	234

AVERAGE POTASSIUM CONTENT NOT AVAILABLE (NA) — but these foods are know to contain more than 230 milligrams per 100 gram portion.

Broadbeans — dry, raw
Buckwheat flour
Carob powder — dry
Pepitas— raw, shelled
Pinon (Pinenut) kernels— raw
Pignolia (Pinenut) kernels— raw
Safflower Seed kernels— raw
Sesame Seeds— hulled, raw
Soya Beans — fresh or sprouted
TVP— hydrated

MAGNESIUM

CONTENT RANGE IN EDIBLE FOODS – FROM THE HIGHEST DOWN

Measured in milligrams per 100 gram portion

Wheat Bran – dry, raw	490	Cheese, Cheddar – natural	45
Wheat Germ – dry, raw	336	Bread – Light Rye	42
Almond kernels – natural, raw	270	Chestnuts – fresh	41
Cashew Nut kernels – raw	267	Okras– raw	41
Soya Beans – dry, raw	265	Prunes – dried	40
Molasses – "Blackstrap"	258	Sunflower Seed kernels – raw	38
Soya Milk – dry	250	Barley – pearled, dry	37
Soya Grits – "low fat"	247	Kohlrabi – raw	37
Yeast, Brewers'	231	Garlic Cloves – raw	36
Buckwheat – raw	229	Bread – Cracked Wheat	35
Brazil Nut kernels – raw	225	Peas, fresh – raw	35
Peanuts – raw, without skins	206		
Hazelnut kernels – raw	184	Currants – dried	34
Sesame Seeds – whole, raw	181	Bananas – ripe, raw	33
Lima Beans – dry, raw	180	Raisins – dried	33
Peanuts – roasted, with skins	175	Beans (long green) – raw	32
Yeast, Torula	165	Chives – raw	32
Millet – whole grain	162	Parsnips– raw	32
Wheat – all varieties	160	Pears – dried	31
Pistachio Nut kernels – raw	158	Sweet Potatoes – raw	31
Rolled Oats – dry	144	Blackberries – raw	30
Pecan Nut kernels – raw	142	Brussel Sprouts – raw	29
Bananas – dehydrated	132	Passionfruit – raw	29
Walnut kernels – raw	131	Rice – Unpolished, boiled	29
Whey Powder– dry	130	Rice – Polished, raw	28
Rye – whole grain	115	Coconut – fresh, milk	28
Flour – Wheat, wholemeal	113	Pork Chops – broiled	27
Pasta, Wholemeal – dry	113	Liver– floured & fried	26
Beet Greens – raw	106	Bacon – grilled	25
Coconut – dry meat shredded	90	Beets – raw	25
Rice – Unpolished, raw	88	Flour – Wheat, white	25
Spinach – raw	88	Loganberries – raw	25
Lentils, Brown – dry, raw	80	Cream from Cows' Milk	25
Bread – Wholemeal	78	Broccoli – raw	24
Bread – Dark Rye	71	Cauliflower – raw	24
Figs – dried	71	Oysters – raw	24
Apricots – dried	62	Carrots – raw	23
Yeast, Bakers' – compressed	59	Leeks – raw	23
Chocolate – Plain, milk	58	Soya Milk – reconstituted	23
Dates, Calif. – natural, dry	58		
Corn, Sweet – raw	48	Apples– dried	22
Pasta, White – dry	48	Bread – White	22
Peaches – dried	48	Celery – raw	22
Coconut – fresh meat	46	Potatoes – raw	22
Avocadoes – all varieties	45		

Continued next page

MAGNESIUM continued

Beef Steak (T-bone) — rare	21	Figs — fresh, raw	20
Broccoli — boiled	21	Raspberries, Red— raw	20
Brussel Sprouts — boiled	21	Turnips — raw	20
Rolled Oats — boiled	21	Watercress — raw	20

AVERAGE MAGNESIUM CONTENT NOT AVAILABLE (NA) — but these foods are known to contain more than 20 milligrams per 100 gram portion.

Apricot nectar — canned
Artichokes, Globe — raw or boiled
Beans (long green) — boiled
Beef Steak (T-bone) —"well done"
Beet Greens — boiled
Bread — Brown
Bread — Mixed Grain
Breadfruit — raw
Bream fish — steamed
Broadbeans — fresh or dry
Buckwheat flour
Bulghur Wheat
Carob Powder — dry
Cheese, Swiss — natural
Chestnuts — dried
Chickpeas (Garbanzos) — dry, raw
Corn Meal — dry
Flounder — baked
Flour — Rye (100%)
Flour — Wheat, White self-raising
Gluten Flour
Ham — deboned, cooked
Haricot Beans — dry or boiled
Kohlrabi — boiled
Lima Beans — boiled

Linseed — whole, raw
Macadamia Nut kernels — raw
Miso
Mung Beans — dry or sprouted
Parsnips — boiled
Peas, fresh — boiled
Pepitas — raw
Pignolia (Pinenut) kernels — raw
Pinon (Pinenut) kernels — raw
Rice Bran — dry, raw
Safflower Seed kernels — raw
Salmon — baked
Scallops — steamed
Semolina — dry
Sesame Seeds — hulled, raw
Swiss Chard—raw or boiled
Soya Beans — fresh or sprouted
Soya Beans — boiled
Soya Grits
Spinach — boiled
Sweet Potatoes — baked or boiled
Tuna — canned in water or oil
TVP — hydrated
Wheat — flaked or rolled
Yeast, Bakers' — dry, active

Vitamins

Vitamins are a group of organic chemical compounds which are largely unrelated insofar as their chemical compositions are concerned. Their relationship derives from their general purpose of facilitating proper nutrition, especially of the major nutrients — proteins, carbohydrates and fats.

The discovery of the role of vitamins in human nutrition is comparatively recent. Only in this century (in 1912) did the chemist, Casimir Funk, first name them. Since then, increasing research has uncovered more and more vitamins, most of which bear code names in alphabetical order of their discovery, or in numerical order if they are regarded as belonging to the B-group of vitamins. Some two dozen vitamins are now known to be factors in the proper assimilation of man's food. Of these, most food analyses have been centered around the vitamins A, B_1, B_2 B_3 and C, for insufficient research has thus far been undertaken on other vitamins in terms of their food origins.

In some publications, vitamin A is listed as either carotene or retinol, or both. For the convenience of guiding the reader to a better understanding of this vitamin in everyday language, this book lists it simply as vitamin A, having calculated all conversions where applicable. Again, some publications give the values for vitamin A, or its components, in International Units or in micrograms — here, we have converted them all to the standard milligram to facilitate better comparisons. Using the generally-accepted ratio of 6000 international units being equivalent to one milligram.

Vitamin A is largely unaffected by heat, as is illustrated by closely related values being given for raw and cooked analyses of the same food. Its major cause of loss is oxidation. Some losses of vitamin A are also caused by prolonged storage.

Likewise, the B-group of vitamins and vitamin C are expressed in milligrams per 100 gram of edible portion of foods. Many vitamins have now been discovered within the group broadly referred to as "B". However, it is only possible to obtain comprehensively researched figures for the first three discovered: Thiamine (B_1), Riboflavin (B_2) and Niacin (B_3). It should be especially noted that of these, vitamin B_1 is the least stable under heat and suffers from greatest loss when foods are exposed to prolonged cooking, as revealed in the comparisons between raw and cooked foods in the general analysis tables.

117

Vitamin C is also known as ascorbic acid. It, too, is diminished by heat. Its richest sources are fruits and vegetables, most of which should be eaten fresh and raw as much as possible to obtain optimum vitamin C. As with all other vitamins, C is measured in milligrams per 100 grams of edible portion. An important aspect of vitamin C in the diet is the manner by which it assists in the metabolism of protein. For this reason, vitamin C-rich foods should always be included in any meal in which protein-rich foods are to be eaten.

The following graduated tables of vitamin contents in foods are consistent with present-day practice wherein only the five aforementioned vitamins are listed.

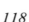

VITAMIN A

Measured in milligrams per 100 gram portion

Cod Liver Oil	29.47	Bananas – dehydrated	.12
Liver– floured & fried	11.18	Peaches – raw	.11
Liver – raw	8.84	Apricot nectar – canned	.10
Peppers, Mature Hot Red – raw	2.17	Tomato Juice – canned	.10
Parsley – raw	1.33	Asparagus – raw or boiled	.09
Carrots – raw	1.25	Oysters – raw	.09
Carrots – boiled	1.17	Peas, fresh – raw	.08
Butter– salted or unsalted	1.0	Pumpkins – raw or boiled	.08
Sweet Potatoes (yellow) – raw	1.0	Soya Beans – fresh	.08
Swiss Chard — raw	.96	Haricot Beans – dry, raw	.07
Spinach – raw	.94	Leeks – raw	.07
Sweet Potatoes –baked in skin	.92	Loquats – raw	.07
Sweet Potatoes (yellow) – boiled	.90	Peas, fresh – boiled	.07
Apricots – dried	.88	Beans (long green) – raw or boiled	.06
Swiss Chard — boiled	.87	Bell Peppers — raw	.06
Spinach – boiled	.85	Chicken – boiled	.06
Mangoes – raw	.80	Leeks – boiled	.06
Eggs (hen) – yolk, raw	.76	Human Milk	.06
Butternut Squash –baked	.74	Okras – raw or boiled	.06
Beet Greens – raw	.69	Watermelons – raw	.06
Chives – raw	.66	Brussel Sprouts – raw or boiled	.05
Butternut Pumpkins – raw	.65	Cheese, Cottage – creamed	.05
Margarine – Cooking	.64	Chicken – fried or roasted	.05
Butternut Squash – boiled	.61	Chocolate – Plain, milk	.05
Beet Greens – boiled	.58	Tangarines – raw	.05
Margarine – Table	.56	Pineapples – raw	.05
Cream from Cows' Milk	.50	Rutabagas – raw	.05
Watercress – raw	.49	Corn, Sweet – raw or boiled	.04
Squash, Winter – raw	.48	Cows' Milk – whole	.04
Squash, Winter – boiled	.47	Goats' Milk – whole	.04
Cheese, Cheddar – natural	.42	Pistachio Nut kernels – raw	.04
Cream Cheese	.41	Plums – raw	.04
Cheese, Swiss – natural	.37	Rutabagas – boiled	.04
Broccoli – raw or boiled	.35	Yogurt from Whole Cows' Milk	.04
Cantaloupes – raw	.34	Avocadoes – all varieties	.03
Tuna – canned in oil	.34	Bananas – ripe, raw	.03
Lettuce – raw	.30	Blackberries – raw	.03
Eggs (hen) – whole, raw	.28	Broadbeans – fresh, raw	.03
Persimmons – raw	.27	Cheese, Ricotta	.03
Apricots – raw	.25	Cherries – raw	.03
Peaches – dried	.21	Cucumbers – whole, raw	.03
Prunes – dried	.18	Gooseberries – raw	.03
Tomatoes – raw	17	Guavas – fresh	.03
Tomatoes – boiled	15	Oranges – raw or juice	.03
Nectarines – raw	.15	Prunes – fresh, raw	.03
Papayas — raw	.13	Salmon – baked	.03

VITAMIN B$_1$ – THIAMINE

CONTENT RANGE IN EDIBLE FOODS – FROM THE HIGHEST DOWN

Measured in milligrams per 100 gram portion

Yeast, Brewers'	15.61	Macadamia Nut kernels – raw	.34
Yeast, Torula	14.01	Chestnuts – dried	.32
Yeast, Bakers' – dry, active	4.17	Peas, fresh – raw	.32
Rice Bran – dry, raw	2.26	Rice – Unpolished, raw	.32
Wheat Germ – dry, raw	2.20	Chickpeas (Garbanzos) – dry, raw	.31
Sunflower Seed kernels – raw	1.96	Liver – raw	.31
"Cornflakes" – dry	1.47	Rye Flour	.30
Pinon (Pinenut) kernels – raw	1.28	Peanuts – roasted, with skins	.29
Soya Milk – dry	1.16	Bulghur Wheat	.28
Soya Beans – dry, raw	1.10	Broadbeans – fresh, raw	.28
Sesame Seeds – whole, raw	.98	Bread – Wholemeal	.27
Brazil Nut kernels – raw	.96	Bread – Cracked Wheat	.27
Peanuts – raw, without skins	.93	Eggs (hen) – yolk, raw	.27
Soya Grits – "low fat"	.87	Liver – floured & fried	.27
Pecan Nut kernels – raw	.86	Garlic Cloves – raw	.25
Soya Flour – "full fat"	.76	Peas, fresh – boiled	.25
Millet – whole grain	.73	Almond kernels – natural, raw	.24
Pork Chops – broiled	.73	Pepitas – raw	.24
Pistachio Nut kernels – raw	.67	Soya Beans – sprouted	.24
Ham – deboned, cooked	.63	Chestnuts – fresh	.22
Pignolia (Pinenut) kernels – raw	.62	Flour–Wheat,White	.22
Buckwheat – raw	.60	Flour – Wheat, White self-raising	.22
Wheat Bran – dry, raw	.60	Peppers, Mature Hot Red – raw	.22
Buckwheat Flour	.58	Bread – Brown	.21
Rolled Oats – dry	.58	Soya Beans – boiled	.21
Wheat, hard red – whole, raw	.57	Artichokes, Jerusalem – raw	.20
Yeast, Bakers' – compressed	.55	Bread – Dark Rye	.20
Flour – Wheat, wholemeal	.51	Bananas – dehydrated	.18
Pasta, Wholemeal – dry	.51	Sesame Seeds – hulled, raw	.18
Bacon – grilled	.50	Bread – Light Rye	.17
Broadbeans – dry, raw	.50	Linseed – whole, raw	.17
Whey Powder – dry	.50	Asparagus – raw	.16
Lima Beans – dry, raw	.48	Asparagus – boiled	.15
Hazelnut kernels – raw	.46	Corn, Sweet – raw	.15
Lentils, Brown – dry, raw	.46	Oysters – raw	.15
Flour – White, fortified	.44	Currants – dried	.14
Haricot Beans – dry, raw	.44	Raisins – dried	.14
Soya Beans – fresh	.44	Bread – White	.13
Cashew Nut kernels – raw	.43	Figs – dried	.13
Rye – Whole grain	.43	Lima Beans – boiled	.13
Wheat, soft – whole, raw	.43	Mung Beans – sprouted	.13
Walnut kernels – raw	.39	Okra – raw	.13
Corn Meal – dry	.38	Parsley – raw	.13
Mung Beans – dry, raw	.38	Semolina – dry	.13
Wheat, soft – flaked & rolled	.36		

Continued next page

Barley — pearled, dry	.12
Chocolate — Plain, milk	.12
Pasta, White — dry	.12
Veal Chops — broiled	.12
Avocadoes — Fuerte	.11
Breadfruit — raw	.11
Corn, Sweet — boiled	.11
Lamb Chops — broiled	.11
Leeks — raw	.11
Soya Milk — reconstituted	.11
Molasses — "Blackstrap"	.11
Spinach — raw	.11
TVP— hydrated	.11
Beef Steak (T-bone)— "well done"	.10
Beet Greens — raw	.10
Broccoli — raw	.10
Brussel Sprouts — raw	.10
Eggs (hen) — whole, raw	.10
Okras — raw	.10
Parsnips — raw	.10
Potatoes — raw	.10
Spinach — raw	.10
Sweet Potatoes — raw	.10
Yams — raw	.10
Broccoli — boiled	.09
Cabbage, Rad — raw	.09
Chocolate — Plain dark	.09
Dates, Calif — natural, dry	.09
Lentils, Brown — boiled	.09
Potatoes — baked or boiled	.09
Prunes — dried	.09
Rice, Unpolished — boiled	.09
Sweet Potatoes — baked or boiled	.09
Watercress — raw	.09

AVERAGE VITAMIN B₁ CONTENT
NOT AVAILABLE (NA) —
but these foods are known to contain
more than .10 milligrams per 100 gram
portion.

Bread — mixed grain
Carob powder — dry
Gluten Flour
Safflower Seed kernels — raw

121

VITAMIN B$_2$ – RIBOFLAVIN

CONTENT RANGE IN EDIBLE FOODS – FROM THE HIGHEST DOWN

Measured in milligrams per 100 gram portion

Yeast, Bakers' – dry, active	5.10	Rye – whole grain	.22
Yeast, Torula	5.06	Broccoli – raw	.21
Yeast, Brewers'	4.28	Mung Beans – dry, raw	.21
Liver – floured & fried	3.80	Avocadoes – average	.21
Liver – raw	3.00	Avocadoes – Fuerte	.20
Whey Powder – dried	2.51	Ham – deboned, cooked	.20
"Cornflakes" – dry	2.10	Peaches – dried	.20
Yeast, Bakers' – compressed	1.73	Soya Beans – sprouted	.20
Wheat Germ – dry, raw	1.30	Spinach – raw or boiled	.20
Almond kernels – natural, raw	.75	Yogurt from Cows' Milk	.20
Cheese, Cheddar – natural	.48	Asparagus – raw	.19
Mushrooms – raw	.44	Broccoli – boiled	.19
TVP – hydrated	.42	Molasses – "Blackstrap"	.19
Eggs (hen) – yolk, raw	.41	Oysters – raw	.19
Cheese, Swiss – natural	.40	Pepitas – raw	.19
Chocolate – Plain, milk	.39	Asparagus – boiled	.18
Chestnuts – dried	.38	Haricot Beans – dry, raw	.18
Millet – whole grain	.38	Lamb Chops – broiled	.18
Peppers, Mature Hot Red – raw	.36	Lima Beans – dry, raw	.18
Soya Grits – "low fat"	.35	Pears – dried	.18
Chicken – fried	.34	Pork Chops – grilled	.18
Soya Milk – dry	.33	Swiss Chard–raw	.18
Bacon – grilled	.31	Apricots – dried	.17
Soya Beans – dry, raw	.31	Broadbeans – fresh, raw	.17
Broadbeans – dry, raw	.30	Buttermilk	.17
Cheese, Cottage – uncreamed	.30	Cows' Milk – whole	.17
Eggs (hen) – whole, raw	.30	Peanuts – raw, without skins	.17
Wheat Bran – dry, raw	.30	Peanuts – roasted, with skins	.17
Eggs (hen) – white, raw	.29	Prunes – dried	.17
Soya Flour – "full fat"	.29	Beef Steak (T-bone) – "rare"	.16
Parsley – raw	.28	Brussel Sprouts – raw	.16
Veal Chops – broiled	.28	Buckwheat – raw	.16
Flour – White, fortified	.26	Cheese, Ricotta	.16
Beef Steak (T-bone) – "well done"	.25	Linseed – whole, raw	.16
Cashew Nut kernels – raw	.25	Peas, fresh – raw	.16
Cheese, Cottage – creamed	.25	Salmon – baked	.16
Rice Bran – dry, raw	.25	Soya Beans – fresh	.16
Bananas – dehydrated	.24	Watercress – raw	.16
Cream Cheese	.24	Beet Greens – boiled	.15
Lentils, Brown – dry, raw	.24	Buckwheat flour	.15
Sesame Seeds – whole, raw	.24	Chicken – boiled or roasted	.15
Pinon (Pinenut) kernels – raw	.23	Chickpeas (Garbanzos) – dry, raw	.15
Sunflower Seed kernels – raw	.23	Chocolate – Plain, dark	.15
Beet Greens – raw	.22	Swiss Chard–boiled	.15
Chestnuts – fresh	.22	Bulghur Wheat	.14

Continued next page

Brussel Sprouts — boiled	.14
Rolled Oats — dry	14
Okras — raw	.14
Peas, fresh — boiled	.14
Whey — liquid	.14
Butternut Squash — baked	.13
Chives — raw	.13
Mung Beans — sprouted	.13
Pecan Nut kernels — raw	.13
Sesame Seeds — hulled, raw	.13
Walnut kernels — raw	.13
Brazil Nut kernels — raw	.12
Corn, Sweet — raw	.12
Figs — dried	.12
Cream from Cows' Milk	.12
Rye Flour	.12
Squash, Winter — raw	.12
Wheat, hard red — whole, raw	.12
Wheat, soft — flaked & rolled	.12
Apples — dried	.11
Bread — Brown	.11
Butternut Squash—raw	.11
Corn Meal — dry	.11
Macadamia Nut kernels — raw	.11
Milk, Goats' — whole	.11
Okras — boiled	.11
Parsnips — raw	.11
Passionfruit — raw	.11
Pumpkins — raw	.11
Wheat, soft — whole, raw	.11

AVERAGE VITAMIN B$_2$ CONTENT NOT AVAILABLE (NA) —
but these foods are known to contain more than .10 milligrams per 100 gram portion.

Carob Powder - dry
Gluten Flour
Hazelnut kernels — raw
Pignolia (Pinenut) kernels — raw
Pistachio Nut kernels — raw
Safflower Seed kernels — raw
Semolina — dry

VITAMIN B3 — NIACIN

CONTENT RANGE IN EDIBLE FOODS — FROM THE HIGHEST DOWN

Measured in milligrams per 100 gram portion

Yeast, Torula	44.4	Bread — Wholemeal	2.6
Yeast, Brewers'	37.9	Bread — Cracked Wheat	2.6
Yeast, Bakers' — dry, active	36.7	Mung Beans — dry, raw	2.6
Rice Bran — dry, raw	29.8	Peas, fresh — raw	2.6
Wheat Bran — dry, raw	21.7	Rye Flour — medium	2.6
Peanuts — raw, without skins	17.4	Soya Grits — "low fat"	2.6
Peanuts — roasted, with skins	16.9	Broadbeans — dry, raw	2.5
Yeast, Bakers' — compressed	16.4	Flounder — baked	2.5
Liver — floured & fried	15.7	Bread — Brown	2.4
Liver — raw	15.0	Oysters — raw	2.4
"Cornflakes" — dry	14.5	Pepitas — raw	2.4
Tuna — canned in water	13.3	Haricot Beans — dry, raw	2.3
Tuna — canned in oil	11.8	Millet — whole grain	2.3
Wheat Germ — dry, raw	9.5	Dates, Calif. — natural, dry	2.2
Chicken — fried	9.1	Lentils, Brown — dry, raw	2.2
Chicken — roasted	7.8	Soya Beans — dry, raw	2.2
Salmon — baked	7.3	Soya Milk — dry	2.2
Veal Chops — broiled	7.1	Soya Flour — "full fat"	2.1
Beef Steak (T-bone)—"well done"	6.7	Chickpeas (Garbanzos) — dry, raw	2.0
Chicken — boiled	6.0	Corn Meal — dry	2.0
Sesame Seeds — whole or hulled	5.4	Lima Beans — dry, raw	2.0
Sunflower Seed kernels — raw	5.4	Molasses — "Blackstrap"	2.0
Peaches — dried	5.3	Peas, fresh — boiled	2.0
Bacon — grilled	5.1	Semolina — dry	2.0
Mushrooms — raw	5.1	Cashew Nut kernels — raw	1.8
Rice — Unpolished, raw	4.6	Corn, Sweet — raw	1.7
Bulghur Wheat	4.5	Figs — dried	1.7
Pinon (Pinenut) kernels — raw	4.5	Potatoes — raw	1.7
Pork Chops — broiled	4.5	Avocadoes — Fuerte	1.6
Buckwheat — raw	4.4	Barley — pearled, dry	1.6
Peppers, Mature Hot Red — raw	4.4	Brazil Nut kernels — raw	1.6
Beef Steak (T-bone) — "rare"	4.3	Broadbeans — fresh, raw	1.6
Wheat, hard red — whole, raw	4.3	Prunes — dried	1.6
Flour — Wheat, wholemeal	4.1	Rice — Polished, raw	1.6
Lamb Chops — broiled	4.1	Rye — whole grain	1.6
Pasta, Wholemeal — dry	4.1	Avocadoes — Average	1.5
Wheat, soft — flaked & rolled	4.1	Pasta, White — dry	1.5
Ham — deboned, cooked	3.7	Passionfruit — raw	1.5
Almond kernels — natural, raw	3.6	Potatoes — baked in skin	1.5
Wheat, soft — whole, raw	3.6	Asparagus — raw	1.4
Flour — White, fortified	3.5	Bread — Light Rye	1.4
Apricots — dried	3.2	Linseed — whole, raw	1.4
Bream fish — steamed	3.0	Pistachio Nut kernels — raw	1.4
Buckwheat flour	2.9	Rice — Unpolished, boiled	1.4
Bananas — dehydrated	2.8	Soya Beans — fresh	1.4

Continued next page

Asparagus — boiled	1.3
Corn, Sweet — boiled	1.3
Flour — Wheat, white	1.3
Flour — Wheat, self-raising	1.3
Macadamia Nut kernels — raw	1.3
Chestnuts — dried	1.2
Guavas — fresh	1.2
Parsley — raw	1.2
Potatoes — boiled in skin	1.2
Broccoli — raw	1.1
Okras — raw	1.1
Artichokes, Globe — raw	1.0
Bread — Dark Rye	1.0
Broccoli — boiled	1.0
Rolled Oats — dry	1.0
Peaches — raw	1.0
Rutabagas — raw	1.0
Walnut kernels — raw	1.0
Zucchinis — raw	1.0

AVERAGE NIACIN CONTENT NOT
AVAILABLE (NA) —
but these foods are known to contain
more than 1.0 milligrams per 100 gram
portion.

Bread — mixed grain
Carob powder — dry
Gluten Flour
Pignolia (Pinenut) kernels — raw
Safflower Seed kernels — raw

VITAMIN C — ASCORBIC ACID

CONTENT RANGE IN EDIBLE FOODS — FROM THE HIGHEST DOWN

Measured in milligrams per 100 gram portion

Peppers, Mature Hot Red — raw	369	Soya Beans — fresh	29
Guavas — fresh	251	Liver — floured & fried	28
Bell Peppers — raw	231	Turnips — raw	28
Currants, Black — raw	209	Rutabagas—boiled	27
Parsley — raw	178	Loganberries — raw	26
Broccoli — raw	117	Peas, fresh — raw	26
Brussel Sprouts — raw	97	Pineapples — raw	26
Broccoli — boiled	92	Radishes — raw	26
Brussel Sprouts — boiled	83	Asparagus — boiled	25
Watercress — raw	74	Onions, young — raw	25
Papayas — raw	64	Passionfruit — raw	24
Cabbage, Red — raw	61	Tomatoes — ripe, raw	24
Kohlrabi — raw	61	Tomatoes — boiled	23
Strawberries — raw	58	Honeydew Melons — raw	23
Cabbage, White — raw	56	Raspberries, Red — raw	23
Chives — raw	56	Blackberries — raw	22
Spinach — raw	56	Cherimoyas — raw	22
Cauliflower — raw	52	Beans (long green) — raw	21
Oranges — peeled, raw	50	Sweet Potatoes (yellow) — raw	21
Orange juice — fresh	49	Okras — boiled	20
Lemons — peeled, raw	47	Peas, fresh — boiled	20
Kohlrabi — boiled	43	Potatoes — raw	20
Cabbage, White — boiled	42	Squash, Summer — raw	20
Lychees — raw	42	Chayotes — raw	19
Cauliflower — boiled	41	Mung Beans — sprouted	19
Mangoes — raw	41	Nectarines — raw	19
Grapefruit — peeled, raw	40	Zucchinis — raw	19
Grapefruit juice — fresh	39	Leeks — raw	18
Lemon juice — fresh	37	Swiss Chard — boiled	18
Limes — peeled, raw	37	Sweet Potatoes (yellow) — baked in skin	17
Currants, Red — raw	36	Tomato juice — canned	17
Rutabagas — raw	36	Turnips — boiled	17
Gooseberries — raw	35	Peaches — dried	16
Liver — raw	34	Potatoes — baked or boiled in skin	16
Asparagus — raw	33	Beet Greens — boiled	15
Spinach — boiled	33	Garlic Cloves — raw	15
Canteloupes	32	Avocadoes — Fuerte	14
Lime juice — fresh	32	Chayotes — boiled	14
Cabbage, Chinese — raw	31	Parsnips — raw	14
Tangarines — peeled, raw	31	Persimmons — raw	14
Beet Greens — raw	30	Avocadoes — Average	13
Broadbeans — fresh, raw	30	Leeks — boiled	13
Okras — raw	30	Lettuce — raw	13
Swiss Chard — raw	30	Soya Beans — sprouted	13
Breadfruit — raw	29		

Continued next page

Artichokes, Globe — raw	12
Beans (long green) — boiled	12
Corn, Sweet — raw	12
Yams — raw	12
Bananas — ripe, raw	11
Butternut Squash — boiled	11
Quinces — raw	11
Squash, Summer — boiled	11
Apples — with peel, raw	10
Apples — dried	10
Apricots — dried	10
Beets — raw	10
Butternut Pumpkins — baked	10
Cucumbers — raw	10
Onions, mature — raw	10
Rhubarb — raw	10
Squash, Winter — raw	10
Sweet Potatoes (yellow) — baked in skin	10

AVERAGE VITAMIN C CONTENT NOT AVAILABLE (NA) —

but this food known to contain more than 10 milligrams per 100 gram portion.

Olives, Green — fresh

For Additional Reference and Reading

Books by David A. Phillips, Ph.D.:

From Soil To Psyche, $3.95

The Soil To Psyche Recipe Book, $3.95
(coauthored with Ann Phillips)

May be purchased in health food stores, book stores, or ordered from Woodbridge Press, P.O. Box 6189, Santa Barbara, CA 93111.

Books by Paavo Airola, Ph.D.:

How To Get Well, $10.95

Are You Confused? $4.95

Hypoglycemia: A Better Approach, $4.95

Everywoman's Book, $14.95

May be purchased in health food stores, book stores, ordered from Woodbridge Press, P.O. Box 6189, Santa Barbara, CA 93111, or directly from: Health Plus Publishers, P.O. Box 22001, Phoenix, AZ 85028.